T0251370

HIV/AIDS Prevention: Current Issues in Community Practice

HIV/AIDS Prevention: Current Issues in Community Practice has been co-published simultaneously as *Journal of Prevention & Intervention in the Community*, Volume 19, Number 1 2000.

The *Journal of Prevention & Intervention in the Community*™ Monographic "Separates" (formerly the *Prevention in Human Services* series)*

For information on previous issues of *Prevention in Human Services*, edited by Robert E. Hess, please contact: The Haworth Press, Inc., 10 Alice Street, Binghamton, NY 13904-1580 USA.

Below is a list of "separates," which in serials librarianship means a special issue simultaneously published as a special journal issue or double-issue *and* as a "separate" hardbound monograph. (This is a format which we also call a "DocuSerial.")

"Separates" are published because specialized libraries or professionals may wish to purchase a specific thematic issue by itself in a format which can be separately cataloged and shelved, as opposed to purchasing the journal on an on-going basis. Faculty members may also more easily consider a "separate" for classroom adoption.

"Separates" are carefully classified separately with the major book jobbers so that the journal tie-in can be noted on new book order slips to avoid duplicate purchasing.

You may wish to visit Haworth's website at . . .

http://www.haworthpressinc.com

. . . to search our online catalog for complete tables of contents of these separates and related publications.

You may also call 1-800-HAWORTH (outside US/Canada: 607-722-5857), or Fax 1-800-895-0582 (outside US/Canada: 607-771-0012), or e-mail at:

getinfo@haworthpressinc.com

HIV/AIDS Prevention: Current Issues in Community Practice, edited by Doreen D. Salina, PhD (Vol. 19, No. 1, 2000). *Helps researchers and psychologists explore specific methods of improving HIV/AIDS prevention research.*

Educating Students to Make-a-Difference: Community-Based Service Learning, edited by Joseph R. Ferrari, PhD, and Judith G. Chapman, PhD (Vol. 18, No. 1/2, 1999). *"There is something here for everyone interested in the social psychology of service-learning." (Frank Bernt, PhD, Associate Professor, St. Joseph's University)*

Program Implementation in Preventive Trials, edited by Joseph A. Durlak and Joseph R. Ferrari, PhD (Vol. 17, No. 2, 1998). *"Fills an important gap in preventive research. . . . Highlights an array of important questions related to implementation and demonstrates just how good community-based intervention programs can be when issues related to implementation are taken seriously." (Judy Primavera, PhD, Associate Professor of Psychology, Fairfield University, Fairfield, Connecticut)*

Preventing Drunk Driving, edited by Elsie R. Shore, PhD, and Joseph R. Ferrari, PhD (Vol. 17, No. 1, 1998). *"A must read for anyone interested in reducing the needless injuries and death caused by the drunk driver." (Terrance D. Schiavone, President, National Commission Against Drunk Driving, Washington, DC)*

Manhood Development in Urban African-American Communities, edited by Roderick J. Watts, PhD, and Robert J. Jagers (Vol. 16, No. 1/2, 1998). *"Watts and Jagers provide the much-needed foundational and baseline information and research that begins to philosophically and empirically validate the importance of understanding culture, oppression, and gender when working with males in urban African-American communities." (Paul Hill, Jr., MSW, LISW, ACSW, East End Neighborhood House, Cleveland, Ohio)*

Diversity Within the Homeless Population: Implications for Intervention, edited by Elizabeth M. Smith, PhD, and Joseph R. Ferrari, PhD (Vol. 15, No. 2, 1997). *"Examines why homelessness is increasing, as well as treatment options, case management techniques, and community intervention programs that can be used to prevent homelessness." (American Public Welfare Association)*

Education in Community Psychology: Models for Graduate and Undergraduate Programs, edited by Clifford R. O'Donnell, PhD, and Joseph R. Ferrari, PhD (Vol. 15, No. 1, 1997). *"An invaluable resource for students seeking graduate training in community psychology . . . [and will] also serve faculty who want to improve undergraduate teaching and graduate programs." (Marybeth Shinn, PhD, Professor of Psychology and Coordinator, Community Doctoral Program, New York University, New York, New York)*

Adolescent Health Care: Program Designs and Services, edited by John S. Wodarski, PhD, Marvin D. Feit, PhD, and Joseph R. Ferrari, PhD (Vol. 14, No. 1/2, 1997). *Devoted to helping practitioners address the problems of our adolescents through the use of preventive interventions based on sound empirical data.*

Preventing Illness Among People with Coronary Heart Disease, edited by John D. Piette, PhD, Robert M. Kaplan, PhD, and Joseph R. Ferrari, PhD (Vol. 13, No. 1/2, 1996). *"A useful contribution to the interaction of physical health, mental health, and the behavioral interventions for patients with CHD. " (Public Health: The Journal of the Society of Public Health)*

Sexual Assault and Abuse: Sociocultural Context of Prevention, edited by Carolyn F. Swift, PhD* (Vol. 12, No. 2, 1995). *"Delivers a cornucopia for all who are concerned with the primary prevention of these damaging and degrading acts." (George J. McCall, PhD, Professor of Sociology and Public Administration, University of Missouri)*

International Approaches to Prevention in Mental Health and Human Services, edited by Robert E. Hess, PhD, and Wolfgang Stark* (Vol. 12, No. 1, 1995). *Increases knowledge of prevention strategies from around the world.*

Self-Help and Mutual Aid Groups: International and Multicultural Perspectives, edited by Francine Lavoie, PhD, Thomasina Borkman, PhD, and Benjamin Gidron* (Vol. 11, No. 1/2, 1995). *"A helpful orientation and overview, as well as useful data and methodological suggestions." (International Journal of Group Psychotherapy)*

Prevention and School Transitions, edited by Leonard A. Jason, PhD, Karen E. Danner, and Karen S. Kurasaki, MA* (Vol. 10, No. 2, 1994). *"A collection of studies by leading ecological and systems-oriented theorists in the area of school transitions, describing the stressors, personal resources available, and coping strategies among different groups of children and adolescents undergoing school transitions." (Reference & Research Book News)*

Religion and Prevention in Mental Health: Research, Vision, and Action, edited by Kenneth I. Pargament, PhD, Kenneth I. Maton, PhD, and Robert E. Hess, PhD* (Vol. 9, No. 2 & Vol. 10, No. 1, 1992). *"The authors provide an admirable framework for considering the important, yet often overlooked, differences in theological perspectives." (Family Relations)*

Families as Nurturing Systems: Support Across the Life Span, edited by Donald G. Unger, PhD, and Douglas R. Powell, PhD* (Vol. 9, No. 1, 1991). *"A useful book for anyone thinking about alternative ways of delivering a mental health service." (British Journal of Psychiatry)*

Ethical Implications of Primary Prevention, edited by Gloria B. Levin, PhD, and Edison J. Trickett, PhD* (Vol. 8, No. 2, 1991). *"A thoughtful and thought-provoking summary of ethical issues related to intervention programs and community research." (Betty Tableman, MPA, Director, Division. of Prevention Services and Demonstration Projects, Michigan Department of Mental Health, Lansing)*

Career Stress in Changing Times, edited by James Campbell Quick, PhD, MBA, Robert E. Hess, PhD, Jared Hermalin, PhD, and Jonathan D. Quick, MD* (Vol. 8, No. 1, 1990). *"A well-organized book. . . . It deals with planning a career and career changes and the stresses involved. " (American Association of Psychiatric Administrators)*

Prevention in Community Mental Health Centers, edited by Robert E. Hess, PhD, and John Morgan, PhD* (Vol. 7, No. 2, 1990). *"A fascinating bird's-eye view of six significant programs of preventive care which have survived the rise and fall of preventive psychiatry in the U.S." (British Journal of Psychiatry)*

Protecting the Children: Strategies for Optimizing Emotional and Behavioral Development, edited by Raymond P. Lorion, PhD* (Vol. 7, No. 1, 1990). *"This is a masterfully conceptualized and edited volume presenting theory-driven, empirically based, developmentally oriented prevention. " (Michael C. Roberts, PhD, Professor of Psychology, The University of Alabama)*

The National Mental Health Association: Eighty Years of Involvement in the Field of Prevention, edited by Robert E. Hess, PhD, and Jean DeLeon, PhD* (Vol. 6, No. 2, 1989). *"As a family life educator* *interested in both the history of the field, current efforts, and especially the evaluation of programs, I find this book quite interesting. I enjoyed reviewing it and believe that I will return to it many times. It is also a book I will recommend to students." (Family Relations)*

A Guide to Conducting Prevention Research in the Community: First Steps, by James G. Kelly, PhD, Nancy Dassoff, PhD, Ira Levin, PhD, Janice Schreckengost, MA, AB, Stephen P. Stelzner, PhD, and B. Eileen Altman, PhD* (Vol. 6, No. 1, 1989). *"An invaluable compendium for the prevention practitioner, as well as the researcher, laying out the essentials for developing effective prevention programs in the community. . . . . This is a book which should be in the prevention practitioner's library, to read, re-read, and ponder." (The Community Psychologist)*

Prevention: Toward a Multidisciplinary Approach, edited by Leonard A. Jason, PhD, Robert D. Felner, PhD, John N. Moritsugu, PhD, and Robert E. Hess, PhD* (Vol. 5, No. 2, 1987). *"Will not only be of intellectual value to the professional but also to students in courses aimed at presenting a refreshingly comprehensive picture of the conceptual and practical relationships between community and prevention." (Seymour B. Sarason, Associate Professor of Psychology, Yale University)*

Prevention and Health: Directions for Policy and Practice, edited by Alfred H. Katz, PhD, Jared A. Hermalin, PhD, and Robert E. Hess, PhD* (Vol. 5, No. 1, 1987). *Read about the most current efforts being undertaken to promote better health.*

The Ecology of Prevention: Illustrating Mental Health Consultation, edited by James G. Kelly, PhD, and Robert E. Hess, PhD* (Vol. 4, No. 3/4, 1987). *"Will provide the consultant with a very useful framework and the student with an appreciation for the time and commitment necessary to bring about lasting changes of a preventive nature." (The Community Psychologist)*

Beyond the Individual: Environmental Approaches and Prevention, edited by Abraham Wandersman, PhD, and Robert E. Hess, PhD* (Vol. 4, No. 1/2, 1985). *"This excellent book has immediate appeal for those involved with environmental psychology . . . likely to be of great interest to those working in the areas of community psychology, planning, and design." (Australian Journal of Psychology)*

Prevention: The Michigan Experience, edited by Betty Tableman, MPA, and Robert E. Hess, PhD* (Vol. 3, No. 4, 1985). *An in-depth look at one state's outstanding prevention programs.*

Studies in Empowerment: Steps Toward Understanding and Action, edited by Julian Rappaport, Carolyn Swift, and Robert E. Hess, PhD* (Vol. 3, No. 2/3, 1984). *"Provides diverse applications of the empowerment model to the promotion of mental health and the prevention of mental illness." (Prevention Forum Newsline)*

Aging and Prevention: New Approaches for Preventing Health and Mental Health Problems in Older Adults, edited by Sharon P. Simson, Laura Wilson, Jared Hermalin, PhD, and Robert E. Hess, PhD* (Vol. 3, No. 1, 1983). *"Highly recommended for professionals and laymen interested in modern viewpoints and techniques for avoiding many physical and mental health problems of the elderly. Written by highly qualified contributors with extensive experience in their respective fields." (The Clinical Gerontologist)*

Strategies for Needs Assessment in Prevention, edited by Alex Zautra, Kenneth Bachrach, and Robert E. Hess, PhD* (Vol. 2, No. 4, 1983). *"An excellent survey on applied techniques for doing needs assessments. . . It should be on the shelf of anyone involved in prevention." (Journal of Pediatric Psychology)*

Innovations in Prevention, edited by Robert E. Hess, PhD, and Jared Hermalin, PhD* (Vol. 2, No. 3, 1983). *An exciting book that provides invaluable insights on effective prevention programs.*

Rx Television: Enhancing the Preventive Impact of TV, edited by Joyce Sprafkin, Carolyn Swift, PhD, and Robert E. Hess, PhD* (Vol. 2, No. 1/2, 1983). *"The successful interventions reported in this volume make interesting reading on two grounds. First, they show quite clearly how powerful television can be in molding children. Second, they illustrate how this power can be used for good ends." (Contemporary Psychology)*

Early Intervention Programs for Infants, edited by Howard A. Moss, MD, Robert E. Hess, PhD, and Carolyn Swift, PhD* (Vol. 1, No. 4, 1982). *"A useful resource book for those child psychiatrists, paediatricians, and psychologists interested in early intervention and prevention." (The Royal College of Psychiatrists)*

Helping People to Help Themselves: Self-Help and Prevention, edited by Leonard D. Borman, PhD, Leslie E. Borck, PhD, Robert E. Hess, PhD, and Frank L. Pasquale* (Vol. 1, No. 3, 1982). *"A timely volume . . . a mine of information for interested clinicians, and should stimulate those wishing to do systematic research in the self-help area." (The Journal of Nervous and Mental Disease)*

Evaluation and Prevention in Human Services, edited by Jared Hermalin, PhD, and Jonathan A. Morell, PhD* (Vol. 1, No. 1/2, 1982). *Features methods and problems related to the evaluation of prevention programs.*

HIV/AIDS Prevention: Current Issues in Community Practice

Doreen D. Salina
Editor

HIV/AIDS Prevention: Current Issues in Community Practice has been co-published simultaneously as *Journal of Prevention & Intervention in the Community*^{TM}, Volume 19, Number 1 2000.

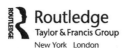

Routledge
Taylor & Francis Group
New York   London

Routledge is an imprint of the
Taylor & Francis Group, an informa business

Transferred to digital printing 2010 by Routledge

Routledge
Taylor and Francis Group
270 Madison Avenue
New York, NY 10016

Routledge
Taylor and Francis Group
2 Park Square
Milton Park, Abingdon
Oxon OX14 4RN

HIV/AIDS Prevention: Current Issues in Community Practice has also been published as *Journal of Prevention & Intervention in the Community,* Volume 19, Number 1 2000.

The development, preparation, and publication of this work has been undertaken with great care. However, the publisher, employees, editors, and agents of The Haworth Press and all imprints of The Haworth Press, Inc., including The Haworth Medical Press and Pharmaceutical Products Press, are not responsible for any errors contained herein or for consequences that may ensue from use of materials or information contained in this work. Opinions expressed by the author(s) are not necessarily those of The Haworth Press, Inc.

Cover design by Thomas J. Mayshock Jr.

The Haworth Press, Inc., 10 Alice Street, Binghamton, NY 13904-1580 USA

Library of Congress Cataloging-in-Publication Data

HIV/AIDS prevention : current issues in community practice / Doreen D. Salina, editor.
     p. cm.
     "Co-published simultaneously as Journal of prevention & intervention in the community, volume 19, number 1, 2000."
     Includes bibliographical references and index.
     ISBN 0-7890-0694-4 (alk. paper)
     1. AIDS (Disease)–Prevention. 2. Community health services. I. Salina, Doreen D.
RA644.A25 H57562 1999
616.97'9205–dc21   99-047991
                                                                      CIP

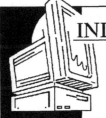

INDEXING & ABSTRACTING

Contributions to this publication are selectively indexed or abstracted in print, electronic, online, or CD-ROM version(s) of the reference tools and information services listed below. This list is current as of the copyright date of this publication. See the end of this section for additional notes.

- *Abstracts of Research in Pastoral Care & Counseling*

- *Behavioral Medicine Abstracts*

- *BUBL Information Service, An Internet-based Information Service for the UK higher education community*

- *Child Development Abstracts & Bibliography*

- *CNPIEC Reference Guide: Chinese National Directory of Foreign Periodicals*

- *EMBASE/Excerpta Medica*

- *Family Studies Database (online and CD/ROM)*

- *HealthPromis*

- *IBZ International Bibliography of Periodical Literature*

- *MANTIS (Manual, Alternative and Natural Therapy) MANTIS is available through three databases vendors: Ovid, Dialog & Datastar. In addition it is available for searching through www.healthindex.com*

- *Mental Health Abstracts (online through DIALOG)*

- *National Center for Chronic Disease Prevention & Health Promotion (NCCDPHP)*

- *National Clearinghouse on Child Abuse & Neglect*

- *NIAAA Alcohol and Alcohol Problems Science Database (ETOH)*

- *OT BibSys*

- *Psychological Abstracts (PsycINFO)*

- *Referativnyi Zhurnal (Abstracts Journal of the All-Russian Institute of Scientific and Technical Information)*

- *RMDB DATABASE (Reliance Medical Information)*

(continued)

- *Social Planning/Policy & Development Abstracts (SOPODA)*

- *Social Work Abstracts*

- *Sociological Abstracts (SA)*

- *SOMED (social medicine) Database*

- *Violence and Abuse Abstracts: A Review of Current Literature on Interpersonal Violence (VAA)*

Special Bibliographic Notes related to special journal issues (separates) and indexing/abstracting:

- indexing/abstracting services in this list will also cover material in any "separate" that is co-published simultaneously with Haworth's special thematic journal issue or DocuSerial. Indexing/abstracting usually covers material at the article/chapter level.
- monographic co-editions are intended for either non-subscribers or libraries which intend to purchase a second copy for their circulating collections.
- monographic co-editions are reported to all jobbers/wholesalers/approval plans. The source journal is listed as the "series" to assist the prevention of duplicate purchasing in the same manner utilized for books-in-series.
- to facilitate user/access services all indexing/abstracting services are encouraged to utilize the co-indexing entry note indicated at the bottom of the first page of each article/chapter/contribution.
- this is intended to assist a library user of any reference tool (whether print, electronic, online, or CD-ROM) to locate the monographic version if the library has purchased this version but not a subscription to the source journal.
- individual articles/chapters in any Haworth publication are also available through the Haworth Document Delivery Service (HDDS).

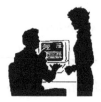

ABOUT THE EDITOR

Doreen D. Salina, PhD, LCP, is Director of Prevention at the Howard Brown Health Center and Assistant Professor of Psychiatry and Behavioral Sciences at Northwestern University Medical School in Chicago, Illinois. Dr. Salina is also in an independent practice as a clinical psychologist. A member of the American Psychological Association in the Divisions of Society for Community Research and Action, Psychology of Women, Health Psychology, and Psychology of Law, Dr. Salina is on the Editorial Board of *Journal of HIV/AIDS Prevention & Education for Adolescents & Children* and is an invited Guest Editor of *Journal of Prevention & Intervention in the Community*, both published by The Haworth Press, Inc. Dr. Salina is the author of over 20 articles and has made over 30 professional presentations focusing on her major areas of interest which include design, implementation, and evaluation of HIV/AIDS and health promotion programs, minority issues, community psychology, behavioral medicine, psychological evaluation and individual children, family treatment, and forensic psychology.

HIV/AIDS Prevention: Current Issues in Community Practice

CONTENTS

Building Collaborative Partnerships to Improve Community-Based HIV Prevention Research: The University-CBO Collaborative Partnership (UCCP) Model

Gary W. Harper

DePaul University

Doreen D. Salina

Northwestern University

SUMMARY. The concept of developing collaborative partnerships with community-based organizations (CBOs) is based on the community psychology perspective of forming reciprocal, nonexploitative partnerships with community members. This perspective has evolved from the empowerment literature which views the community psychologist as a collaborator with community members who participate in all aspects of an intervention and evaluation. This article presents a conceptual model of effective university-CBO partnerships, with emphasis on HIV prevention research. A six stage model is presented, with emphasis on the beginning stages of developing collaborations with AIDS related CBOs. These stages are: 1. Selecting a potential CBO partner; 2. Developing a reciprocal relationship; 3. Deciding on a research question; 4. Conducting the research/evaluation; 5. Analyzing and interpreting the data; and 6. Dissemination. Barriers to effective collaboration are discussed. These barriers include having different goals, relationships that are not perceived as mutually beneficial, unfamiliarity with cultural

[Haworth co-indexing entry note]: "Building Collaborative Partnerships to Improve Community-Based HIV Prevention Research: The University-CBO Collaborative Partnership (UCCP) Model." Harper, Gary W., and Doreen D. Salina. Co-published simultaneously in *Journal of Prevention & Intervention in the Community* (The Haworth Press, Inc.) Vol. 19, No. 1, 2000, pp. 1-20; and: *HIV/AIDS Prevention: Current Issues in Community Practice* (ed: Doreen D. Salina) The Haworth Press, Inc., 2000, pp. 1-20. Single or multiple copies of this article are available for a fee from The Haworth Document Delivery Service [1-800-342-9678, 9:00 a.m. - 5:00 p.m. (EST). E-mail address: getinfo@haworthpressinc.com].

1

norms, and power differentials between university based researchers and CBO staff and community members. Strategies to avoid these potential problems are presented. *[Article copies available for a fee from The Haworth Document Delivery Service: 1-800-342-9678. E-mail address: getinfo@haworthpressinc.com <Website: http://www.haworthpressinc.com>]*

KEYWORDS. HIV prevention, community psychology, collaborative partnership

INTRODUCTION

Community psychologists have been dedicated to improving the health and well being of individuals and communities for well over thirty years (Bennet, Anderson, Cooper, Hassol, Klein, & Rosenblum, 1966; Heller, Price, Reinharz, Riger, Wandersman, & D'Aunno, 1984; Rappaport, 1977). One major focus of community psychology which has differentiated it from related fields such as clinical, social and organizational psychology has been a focus on the prevention of negative physical and mental health outcomes (Heller et al., 1984; Kelly, 1990). In their attempts to create more effective prevention interventions, many community psychologists have worked in close collaboration with community members and community agencies during most phases of their program development and implementation. Although some early efforts in community psychology placed the psychologist in the role of an "expert advisor," there has been significant movement toward building more equal partnerships with community-based organizations (CBOs). When these efforts are successful, the strengths and abilities of both the university researcher and the CBO are combined in a synergistic fashion to create community programs that are acceptable, feasible, and effective.

The concept of developing collaborative partnerships with CBOs is also broadly based in the community psychology perspective of developing an empowerment research agenda whereby individuals who were previously considered research subjects or participants become research collaborators (Rapoport, 1985; Rappaport, 1987, 1990; Serrano-Garcia, 1990; Zimmerman & Rappaport, 1988; Zimmerman, Israel, Schulz, & Checkoway, 1992). This perspective more specifically follows from the practice of empowerment evaluation (Fetterman, 1994, 1996; Fetterman, Kaftarian, & Wandersman, 1996; Zimmerman, in press). In empowerment collaborations the evaluation process is designed to allow individuals, organizations or communities to actively participate in all steps of an evaluation (Fetterman, 1996) with the community psychologist's role shifting from one of expert and counselor to one of collaborator and facilitator (Zimmerman, in press). Therefore, establishing and maintaining collaborative partnerships with CBOs are essential components to an empowerment agenda.

University-CBO Collaborative Partnerships

Prudent research methodologies in community psychology require a thorough understanding of the contexts and structures of specific communities. In order to fully understand these mechanisms and processes, researchers must venture outside of traditional university-based settings and observe and interact with individuals in their community environments. Unfortunately, this mission may be difficult to complete if the researcher is not familiar with the social framework of the communities in which their populations of interest function. In addition, individuals from economically disadvantaged and marginalized communities may be especially suspicious of university researchers who they perceive wish only to observe them and do not provide tangible services to the members of their community. Gomez and Goldstein (1996) have posited that key differences between CBOs and universities with regard to money, ownership, rigor, and time (MORT) may also contribute toward the historical mistrust between these two entities. One effective solution is for researchers to work collaboratively with CBOs that are already integrated into the fabric of their population's social environment. These CBOs are already established within their respective communities and their direct participation in the evaluation component provides overt legitimization of evaluation activities to the recipients. This synergistic union of practical "front line" experience with knowledge of theory and evaluation skills can greatly improve both the services delivered and the quality of data collected. This joint collaboration allows accurate evaluation of the programs of the CBO, which in turn may be utilized to improve the efficacy and delivery of the service.

While researchers and CBOs may have the common goal of social action and change, forming and maintaining collaborative relationships between university-based researchers and CBOs can be challenging at times. Since the primary focus of researchers is to scientifically collect data while the primary goal of the CBO is to provide direct services, the specific methods of achieving these goals may sometimes conflict. Unfortunately, this "science vs. service" dilemma sometimes results in CBOs becoming disillusioned with university involvement, especially when CBO staff experience the researcher as exploiting the community for scientific and personal gain. This occurs primarily when the relationship is not perceived as reciprocal and mutually beneficial. In addition, since the organizational cultures of CBOs and universities are often quite different, unintentional misunderstandings may occur that create barriers and tensions that impede collaborative efforts. Researchers and CBO staff who are not familiar with the other's cultural norms are less effective, and negative stereotypes of each other may develop or be reinforced. Additional barriers to collaborative partnerships may include political issues within the community, issues of systems change in the delivery of social services, and institutional constraints that are in effect within the university (McHale & Lerner, 1996).

There is increasing awareness of the benefits of forming more collaborative partnerships between universities and CBOs in order to address specific social issues (e.g., Binson, Harper, Grinstead, & Haynes-Sanstad, 1997; Gomez & Goldstein, 1996; McHale & Lerner, 1996; Ostrom, Lerner, & Freel, 1995; Paine-Andrews, Fawcett, Richter, Berkley, Williams, & Lopez, 1996; Small, 1996). Some of these models have focused on the broad categories of steps that are included in the collaborative process such as Ostrom et al.'s (1995) DICE model. DICE includes the four components of: (a) evaluation design, (b) data collection, (c) data analysis, and (d) use of findings to promote community change. Others have presented more ecological and/or interactive models such as Small's (1996) Collaborative Research Model that emphasizes the reciprocal interactional relationships among citizens, knowledge, and researchers. In addition, Binson et al.'s (1997) Technology and Information Exchange Model which is a model for technology and information exchange has received serious attention and application. This model uses a mix of information and interaction in an effort to integrate practice among researchers, service providers, and policymakers, and to inform the public. Less attention has been addressed to the early aspects of community collaboration, with the resulting effect that well designed interventions have been less effective due to resistance from community participants. It is our premise that by conducting an early in-depth assessment of the commonalities and differences between the university and community perspective, many of the barriers encountered may be minimized or avoided to enrich the actual collaboration.

The University-CBO Collaborative Partnership (UCCP) Model

In the paper we present a six stage model to address the interactional processes that occur while developing and maintaining collaborative research partnerships between universities and CBOs. This model differs from those previously discussed in that it has a strong emphasis on the specific processes that occur during the beginning stages of developing a collaborative relationship. Table 1 presents the six stages of the model along with critical questions that should be addressed at each stage. This paper emphasizes the first two stages related to identifying an agency and building a collaborative partnership. We focus on these stages since without successful navigation through these, later efforts are generally compromised. These first stages are especially important when attempting to form collaborations with HIV/AIDS service organizations since HIV infection is intimately connected with a myriad of social, political, religious, psychological, and medical issues and controversies. Researchers who are considering forming a collaborative partnership with an HIV-related CBO need to spend extra time exploring how these factors are manifested for the specific community and identify potential barriers to successful implementation of the program. Without this preliminary work, the feasibility of such a relationship is questionable and the potential costs may outweigh the potential benefits for both the CBO and the researchers.

TABLE 1. UNIVERSITY-CBO COLLABORATIVE PARTNERSHIP (UCCP) MODEL

1. Selecting a Potential CBO Partner.

    Who is serving the population of interest? What services do they provide?
    Does the CBO have the desire to be involved in a research project? Do they have the time and resources?
    Do the researchers have anything to offer the CBO? Can this be both a collaborative and reciprocal relationship?

2. Developing a Reciprocal Relationship.

    How do the priorities and goals of CBOs and universities differ?

How does the language and culture of CBOs and universities differ?

How does the work space and environment of CBOs and universities differ?

Who is responsible for each component? Do we need a contract?

3. Deciding on a Research/Evaluation Question.

What do we both want to accomplish? Can we do this with this question?

Who will truly benefit from the outcome?

Can the project be completed given the resources that are available and if so, can it be done in a collaborative manner?

4. Conducting the Research/Evaluation.

Who will recruit and how will they do it? How do the criteria for inclusion in the study differ from the criteria for the receiving of services? Is the staff following the inclusion/exclusion criteria? If not, why?

How do the researchers guarantee the quality of data collection? How often should the researchers visit the CBO? How often should the CBO visit the university?

How does one control for CBO staff burnout?

5. Analyzing and Interpreting the Data.

How involved should the CBO be in deciding how to analyze the data?

Who should interpret the findings? What about conflicts in data interpretation?

Do these analyses and interpretations meet the needs of the CBO and the university?

6. Disseminating the Findings.

Where should these findings be published? Authorship?

How do the researchers disseminate the findings to other community members in a form they can understand and use to improve services/policy?

What can the researchers leave with the CBO and the community at large after the project is terminated? Was the relationship truly reciprocal? What can be improved?

Selecting a Potential CBO Partner

Before a researcher decides to attempt to form a collaborative partnership with a specific CBO, it is essential that several important questions be addressed, as they are likely to impact the effectiveness of the collaboration. For the researchers, level of comfort with both the targeted community and the people impacted with HIV/AIDS and their lifestyle behaviors needs to be addressed and clarified. Since the norms, language and belief systems of the specific community may be different than those of the researcher and almost surely are different from the university culture, strategies that address these differences are necessary, not only for the research team, but in anticipation of the responses from CBO staff. In addition, many of the populations who are most impacted by HIV (e.g., injection drug users, gay men, low-income ethnic minorities) are marginalized members of American society. Individuals in these communities are considered marginalized because of some known or perceived characteristic or behavior that places them outside normative standards of mainstream culture. The level of familiarity and understanding the researcher displays with community members will impact on the willingness of the CBO staff to participate in research efforts. Therefore, a university researcher who is interested in forming collaborations with HIV/AIDS-related CBOs must explore any personal prejudices that s/he may have toward those at-risk for or living with HIV.

The first action to be taken when building a collaborative partnership with a CBO is finding the most appropriate CBO partner. The decisions that are made at this phase of the process will have major ramifications for the eventual success or failure of the collaboration. If there is a good match or fit between the university researcher and CBO, the relationship will often be synergistic, and the science and service outcomes will be substantial. If there is not a good fit, the collaborative effort can become laborious, and neither the CBO nor the researcher, and more importantly the population of interest, will benefit. The researchers must identify the various organizations which serve his/her particular population of interest and which would benefit from the collaboration.

The task of finding a CBO partner in the field of HIV may be different than with other areas of collaboration due to the sociopolitical nature of HIV and the stigma surrounding the disease. The level of distrust for university researchers may be especially high due to earlier work which has sometimes been used to label and stigmatize people with HIV/AIDS. The researcher is best served by gathering information about the CBO prior to approaching the CBO staff. Most CBOs have printed materials describing their agency services and annual or quarterly summaries/reports, both of which can be easily obtained with a brief phone call. The city's Department of Public Health can also be an excellent resource, especially when the city has a division specifically focused on or including HIV/AIDS issues. Many urban environments have city-specific AIDS Foundations (e.g., AIDS Foundation of Chicago, San Francisco AIDS Foundation) and these can be excellent resources. In addition, most gay/lesbian/bisexual-specific newspapers and other publications contain listings of HIV/AIDS-related organizations. Information that is particularly valuable is that which presents information about previous or ongoing research interventions. The identification of other researchers who have been involved in research projects with the specific CBO or the targeted population provides a useful context within which to understand attitudes towards researchers. In addition, if the previous researchers have first hand knowledge about the particular CBO, they may be able to identify potential concerns or barriers that the researchers can be prepared to address.

The search for a CBO may also extend beyond those organizations that only provide HIV-specific services. This is especially the case when dealing with a highly specific population or one that is not typically viewed as being a target only of HIV/AIDS services. In addition, researchers working in more rural or suburban communities may find a paucity of HIV-specific agencies. Many community health centers, community mental health centers, and community substance abuse treatment centers have divisions or programs that are focused on providing HIV-related prevention and/or treatment services. Some CBOs that are focused on providing services to a specific population (e.g., inner-city ethnic-minority youth) may also have programs that provide HIV services. General information about these organizations may be obtained from the local Department of Public Health, Department of Mental Health, and/or Department of Alcohol and Substance Abuse, and more specific information about these organizations can typically be obtained through the solicitation of printed materials before actually meeting with the staff.

There are several types of basic information that are important to gather before making the decision to approach a particular CBO. The first is to clarify what population(s) the agency serves and the specific services provided. Also, it is useful to know where the agency is located, where the various services are delivered, and how many individuals receive services each year. Knowing the relative size of the CBO may give the researcher information about the CBO's potential to work in a collaborative research capacity. In addition, the researcher should ascertain whether or not the CBO has the resources to collaboratively participate in a research project. These resources may include components such as the people to conduct the research/evaluation and time allotted for these individuals to actually work on the project instead of their usual tasks/duties. Other resources include physical space to engage in the various project related activities, computers or other types of mechanical supports that may be needed for the project, and financial resources or the ability/desire to write grants to obtain needed funds.

Developing a Reciprocal Relationship

Once the researcher has identified a potential CBO partner, s/he must approach the CBO to assess their level of interest in forming a collaborative partnership. This initial contact can be very important since CBOs that have not previously considered university involvement may easily dismiss a researcher if the researcher presents him/herself in a manner that violates community norms, indicates a power differential, or suggests any type of bias or stereotypical beliefs. Identification of the appropriate staff member is crucial, since the initial contact may be the last if the staff member contacted does not have the authority to agree or decline an invitation to participate. This phone contact should provide the CBO contacts with enough information to decide whether or not they want to meet the researcher, with the understanding that an agreement to meet does not translate into an agreement to participate in the collaboration.

It is often preferable to have this initial meeting at the CBO's site, as this gesture sends several positive messages to the CBO. It lets the CBO know that the researcher is willing to leave the protected domain of the university and visit the community. This may be an especially important message when the CBO is located in a community or part of the city that is economically distressed and that is often not frequented by individuals other than those who reside there. Even if the research-er is someone who has worked in various communities for years, the CBO may not be aware of this and may have preconceived notions of university researchers and assume that the researcher is not connected to or familiar with the community of interest. Going out to the CBO site instead of having the CBO staff visit the university also helps to balance any initial perceived power differential. It also allows the researcher the opportunity to meet with several individuals from the CBO and maximize the potential for consensus about important as-pects of the collaboration.

Prior to the meeting, the researcher may want to send any relevant materials to the CBO so that the agency can have some additional knowledge of the researcher and his/her work. This may include items such as a curriculum vita, HIV-related and CBO-related publications and/or presentations, and curriculum guides for any previous HIV prevention programs. The researcher should send this information far enough in advance so that the agency can distribute the materials to all interested personnel prior to the meeting.

Upon meeting, both the researcher and the CBO begin the process of deciding whether or not the two parties can form a collaborative partnership and what questions will be answered from the research endeavor. In order to have a mutually beneficial and productive work-ing relationship, both parties may need to first explore some of their basic philosophical issues regarding HIV prevention and treatment. If there are serious differences between the researcher's views of "ap-propriate" HIV prevention and treatment services and the CBO's views of such activities, it will make the project more difficult and may even prohibit each partner from being able to form a truly collab-orative relationship.

These discrepancies occur more in the HIV field than in other areas of prevention and intervention since HIV/AIDS is still a relatively new topic of research. Clear and mutually agreed upon definitions of risk and guidelines for prevention and treatment do not always exist. Dis-agreements often arise around issues such as (a) the degree of risk associated with certain sexual activities (e.g., oral sex); (b) the ap-propriateness of harm reduction vs. treatment and abstinence for injec-tion drug users; (c) the use of alternative therapies such as Chinese herbs, cannabis, or acupuncture; (d) the acceptance of doctor-assisted suicide. All of these issues may not be addressed in the very first meeting, but this is a good place to begin the dialogue on potentially ambiguous areas so that controversies and disagreements do not arise in the middle of the collaborative effort. It is best to learn about philosophical discrepancies initially then negotiate a specific compromise if necessary before the collaborative effort is implemented.

If the CBO is focused on working with populations which have little power or control over their life circumstances, such as youth who are homeless or adults with chronic/persistent mental illness, the researcher and CBO staff may need to discuss their views on recruitment and retention of participants. The researcher and CBO may have conflicting views of how issues such as consent and treatment should be handled with these individuals, and even though both parties do not have to share the same exact opinions, they should not have diametrically opposed positions.

Once these areas are addressed, the CBO staff and researchers are prepared to develop the specifics of the collaboration. One may expect that there will be a wide range of expertise within both the CBO and the specific community. Informal methods of assessing these resources may provide more information than simply reading about these individuals or about the CBO. It is important for the researcher to make several visits to the CBO to learn about the program specific activities as well as the day-to-day activities of the agency as a whole and the people that will be involved in the research/evaluation project. Attention should be paid to the work environment, the language and interactional styles, the various demands put on each staff member, and other general differences between the "academic world" and the "CBO world." It is important that the researcher also use this time to let the people in the agency begin to learn more about him/her, keeping in mind that the information flow should be bi-directional.

During the initial meetings it is also beneficial to assess the CBO's knowledge of research and program evaluation. If the CBO is not familiar with these activities, the researcher may need to provide in house training for CBO members about the practical aspects of developing and implementing various evaluation designs, as well as the differences between research and program evaluation.[1] This is consistent with empowerment theory as the researcher provides the community members with requisite skills to maintain and develop additional programs.

Both parties should also discuss their priorities regarding the research and/or evaluation projects early in the collaborative process. This is where the "science vs. service" dilemma discussions may begin and both members may work toward the resolution of this potential conflict. In addition, the early identification of what commodities and services will be exchanged during this collaboration should be discussed since this will facilitate the development of a mutually beneficial collaborative relationship. Both partners should be in agreement as to the roles and responsibilities of each member. A mutually drafted contract is beneficial for many partnerships so as to avert future discrepancies regarding initial agreements.

Deciding on a Research/Evaluation Question

As the collaborative partnership develops, both parties must agree upon a mutually beneficial research and/or evaluation question that can be answered by implementing a practical research/evaluation design. The researcher should assure that the design is scientifically sound, and the CBO should assure that the design is one which will be feasible given the agency's resources, and acceptable and beneficial to the population of interest. It is crucial that both the researcher and the CBO spend time critically analyzing the research question since the practicality of the question can, in large part, determine the success or failure of the collaborative endeavor. When potential designs are being considered, it may be beneficial to create timelines for each of the required tasks along with an estimation of the amount of money and person-hours required to accomplish all of the desired goals. All of those involved in this process should be as realistic as possible, and appropriate consultations should be made when ambiguities exist.

In addition to being scientifically sound, feasible, and acceptable to the population of interest, the design should be one that utilizes the talents and expertise of both the university researcher and all of those involved from the CBO. It should have the potential of being conducted in a collaborative manner, and not rely too heavily on any one partner for successful completion. The question and subsequent design should also ultimately answer a research or evaluation question that will prove to not only be mutually beneficial to the university researcher and CBO, but also the population that the program is being designed to serve.

It is important that the CBO staff involved in the research/evaluation feel a sense of shared ownership for the project so that they will put forth their best effort in conducting their agreed-upon activities. This stage offers an excellent opportunity to have various CBO staff members join in the process. Front-line workers often have a more accurate perception of the acceptability and feasibility of the project for the intended audience than the CBO's director or CEO. Various staff members may also have creative and innovative ideas of how to serve the population since they are the ones spending the majority of their time interacting with the people that the program is intended to serve. It is much more empowering to include those who will be implementing a significant portion of the intervention or research/evaluation during this early developmental stage than to wait until the project has already been developed and then "assign" tasks to the workers. This inclusion widens the scope of the collaborative nature of the project and typically results in an improved research/evaluation design and a smoother running of the project, since the workers feel a sense of shared ownership and commitment to the success of the program.

Conducting the Research/Evaluation

This stage may vary greatly depending on the CBO's prior experience with research/evaluation and the investment of the CBO project staff who will be involved in the project. For those CBOs who have little to no prior research/evaluation experience, the researcher may need to spend some time educating staff about essential components of research and evaluation. It is crucial to relate to the CBO workers the importance of underlying aspects of research/evaluation that the researcher may take for granted, such as the need for consistency/replicability, objectivity, and accurate documentation. In doing this the researcher should be sensitive to the culture and philosophy of the CBO and find ways to make the information easily understood and accessible. The researcher should also strive to present the information in an interactive manner that helps to reinforce the workers' sense of involvement in the project. Strict didactic sessions that create power differentials between the university researcher and the CBO workers should be avoided since they may lead to feelings that the relationship will not be collaborative and a general sense of disenchantment with the research/evaluation project.

The members of the collaborative partnership will need to make collective decisions regarding the selection of clients who will be involved in the research/evaluation project. This task may be less complicated in the case of evaluations where the goal is to assess either the process or outcome of an already existing program. In this situation it may be that all clients or a subset of the clients who receive their usual services will be involved in the project. In the case of a specific research project where participant selection may be more controlled, a set of clearly defined inclusion/exclusion criteria as well as a method for recruitment of participants will need to be developed. It is crucial that all of those involved in the recruitment process be clear as to proper procedures and that these workers are willing and able to meet the demands of the research protocol. Spot checks may need to be conducted to assure that the criteria are being adhered to throughout the life of the study. However, given that the CBO's primary directive is service delivery, the researcher must be prepared for instances where scientific rigor may need to be modified because of individual participants' acute needs. The researcher need not despair, however, for if such instances are prepared for, they provide important qualitative information about the specific population. This early preparation by the researcher will also communicate an understanding to the CBO staff that both parties view the need of the participant as primary.

For those staff who may be involved in the implementation of a new intervention, appropriate training will need to be conducted. Interaction-based training sessions with immediate feedback are useful in helping those involved to acquire the new skills that they will need to implement the program. Once the program is in effect, fidelity checks should be conducted to assure that the program is being delivered in an appropriate and consistent manner. Regular meetings with the program staff should be conducted so that potential barriers to appropriate program implementation can be addressed. Some CBO workers may not independently approach the university researcher with implementation difficulties, but if a regular forum for the open discussion of such issues is provided, s/he may feel more comfortable in addressing such issues.

Once the research/evaluation project has begun and is in full operation, some university researchers make the mistake of drastically decreasing their contact with the CBO. Although the amount of time actually spent at the agency may decrease somewhat, the researcher should still make relatively frequent visits to the CBO and/or the program implementation sites. This not only helps the researcher to stay informed as to the progress of the project, but also sends a strong message to the CBO that the researcher is truly a collaborative partner and is committed to the success of the program. The researcher should be careful not to make the visits appear as if they are times when the workers are being scrutinized or monitored, but casual visits to observe and appreciate the progress that is being made. In order to avoid staff burnout, it is also helpful to provide periodic group incentives such as pizza parties and/or picnics during paid staff hours. This gives all of those involved in the project a chance to socialize and to spend paid time away from the program participants. This is especially necessary in the HIV field since the emotional intensity of the work can be draining.

Analyzing and Interpreting the Data

Consistent with proper research design, the primary questions to be answered must be identified prior to the implementation of the program. However, in applied research, other questions of interest to one or both parties will generally arise. If not conducted in a collaborative manner, the data analysis and interpretation stage can cause conflict in relationships that were heretofore harmonious. Given limited evaluation resources, all questions may not be able to be analyzed, and differences of opinion may impede the collaborative effort. These conflicts may focus on what the most crucial questions to answer are, or on differences about the interpretations and implications of the findings. Another crucial issue that may arise at this stage is ownership of the data. Each collaborative partnership will need to struggle with solutions to these issues, and it is prudent to discuss these at the outset of the collaborative partnership and to clearly outline roles and responsibilities in the initial contract so as to decrease later ambiguities and conflicts. Specific uses of the data for both partners complete the collaborative effort. Data may be used for new funding efforts by either party to demonstrate impact of existing programs or to highlight an underfunded problem affecting the community.

The level of involvement that the members of the CBO have in the data analysis process will depend partly on their level of interest and expertise in data analysis. If the CBO staff have only a basic level of understanding regarding data analytic techniques, the researcher can present appropriate information in a manner that is easily understood.

The researcher should be careful not to use so much statistical jargon that the members of the CBO are too intimidated to ask questions or to challenge statistical suggestions. The connection between the initial research/evaluation questions and the data analytic plan should be explored, and all members should assure that the information gained will be practical and useful.

Data interpretation can be a delicate issue. The interpretation that is placed upon the data generated from the project will influence society's views of the population of interest. Unfortunately, there exists a history of scientific data being used to promote and maintain negative stereotypes of various marginalized and stigmatized populations. Many communities are aware of these injustices and thus may be especially sensitive to the manner in which the data are being interpreted. Additional concerns may arise when the researcher is not a member of the population of interest. If there are no members of the community working on the interpretation of the data, the researcher and CBO should attempt to involve representative members who can assist the team in making accurate and sensitive interpretations. These members can be recruited through the community mechanism, or a student volunteer can become involved. The interpretation process should be an iterative one that involves a voicing of multiple perspectives, and an attempt should be made to reach consensus on these sensitive issues.

Both partners in the collaboration must work together to recognize preconceived stereotypes that may exist during data interpretations as they attempt to understand the obtained results. This may be difficult at times because of emotional ties to the data that may develop as a result of large expenditures of time and energy that have gone into the data collection. Ambiguities may also arise when members who are not familiar with data analysis are confused about the implications of particular findings and limits about the generalizability of the data. The researcher must strive to present an unbiased view of the data analytic findings so that the CBO and other members of the population can form their own conclusions. All involved in the interpretive process should be acutely aware of the potential impact that their interpretations may have on the population that they are attempting to serve. This multidimensional perspective will likely provide a richness of interpretation that would generally be lacking.

Dissemination

Although academic researchers may traditionally think of publications in peer-reviewed journals as the primary form of dissemination, this venue may not be of interest to those working in a CBO. Since the partnership is collaborative, the researcher and CBO will need to agree how and where the information from the project will be disseminated. The researcher may need to be open to disseminating information in non-traditional academic forums such as agency/coalition newsletters, service provider workshops and conferences, or agency-generated pamphlets and brochures.

When preparing the data for non-academic audiences, each member of the partnership will need to use their areas of expertise to assure that the pertinent information gets translated into a form that may result in improved services and policies for the population of interest. Presentations for community audiences should avoid technical jargon and non-applied information. It is also helpful to include members of the population of interest in this process so that the material is sensitive to the culture and language of the community.

Regardless of whether data dissemination is occurring through academic avenues or through agency publications, the issue of authorship will need to be discussed. Since the partnership is collaborative, appropriate authorship credit should be given to those individuals intimately involved in the process, regardless of their educational background and/or affiliation. It is helpful to decide on authorship issues as a dissemination plan is being developed, not after the materials/articles have already been produced. Some partnerships may want to make global authorship rules (e.g., certain key individuals will be on all publications/presentations) at the outset of the collaboration and include that in their initial contract or agreement.

Just as data dissemination through peer-reviewed journals may assist the researcher in obtaining tenure/promotion or future research grant funding, dissemination for the CBO may assist in obtaining future funding for services. This not only results in expanded and improved services for the population of interest, but also increased employment opportunities for agency staff. The receipt of such future funds will help newly developed or expanded prevention/service programs to become self-sustaining. The ultimate outcomes of thoroughly evaluated and improved services, along with future funding to expand

and maintain services are some of the primary benefits to collaboration for CBOs.

As the collaborative partnership nears termination, it is beneficial for the researcher to reflect on his/her relationship with the CBO and to critically examine whether or not the relationship was truly reciprocal and mutually beneficial. If this balance has not been achieved, the researcher may extend the relationship until s/he can work with the CBO so that the organization and the people served by the organization are left with new valuable resources. If the researcher does not work to achieve this reciprocity, the negative stereotypes of universities exploiting CBOs to collect data will continue to be reinforced and this may have far reaching effects with regard to future researchers' ability to collaborate with CBOs. A mutual termination of the relationship where all members perceive the experience as a true reciprocal partnership provides both quantitative and qualitative support for the occurrence of an effective collaborative effort.

NOTE

1. There are several free publications that the researcher may want to order which offer this information, including: (a) *Prevention Plus III* (Linney & Wandersman, 1991), published by the Office for Substance Abuse Prevention and distributed by the National Clearinghouse for Alcohol and Drug Information (1-800-729-6686); (b) The *NMHA Guide to Establishing Community-Based Prevention Programs* (McElhaney, 1995), published by the National Mental Health Association (703-684-7722); and (c) *Evaluating HIV/AIDS Prevention Programs in Community-Based Organizations* (National Community AIDS Partnership, 1993) published by the National Community AIDS Partnership (202-429-2820).

REFERENCES

Bennett, C. C., Anderson, L. S., Cooper, S., Hassol, L., Klein, D. C., & Rosenblum, G. (Eds.) (1966). *Community psychology: A report of the Boston conference on the education of psychologists for community mental health.* Boston: Boston University Press.

Binson, D., Harper, G., Grinstead, O., & Haynes-Sanstad, K. (1997). The Center for AIDS Prevention Studies collaboration program: An alliance of AIDS scientists and community-based organization. In P. Nyden, A. Figert, M. Shibley, & D. Burrows (Eds.). *Building community: Social science in action.* Thousand Oaks: Pine Forge Press.

Fetterman, D. M. (1996). Empowerment evaluation: An introduction to theory and practice. In D. M. Fetterman, S. J. Kaftarian, & A. Wandersman (Eds.). *Empowerment evaluation: Knowledge and tools for self-assessment and accountability.* Thousand Oaks: Sage Publications.

Fetterman, D. M., Kaftarian, S. J., & Wandersman, A. (Eds.) (1996). *Empowerment evaluation: Knowledge and tools for self-assessment and accountability.* Thousand Oaks: Sage Publications.

Gomez, C. A., & Goldstein, E. (1996). The HIV prevention evaluation initiative: A model for collaborative and empowerment evaluation. In D. M. Fetterman, S. J. Kaftarian, & A. Wandersman (Eds.). *Empowerment evaluation: Knowledge and tools for self-assessment and accountability.* Thousand Oaks: Sage Publications.

Heller, K., Price, R. H., Reinharz, S., Riger, S., Wandersman, A., & D'Aunno, T. A. (1984). *Psychology and community change* (2nd Ed.). Chicago: The Dorsey Press.

Kelly, J. G. (1990). Changing contexts and the field of community psychology. *American Journal of Community Psychology, 18,* 769-792.

McHale, S. M., & Lerner, R. M. (1996). University-community collaborations on behalf of youth. *Journal of Research on Adolescence, 6,* 1-8.

Ostrom, C. W., Lerner, R. M., & Freel, M. A. (1995). Building the capacity of youth and families through university-community collaborations: The Development-In-Context Evaluation (DICE) Model. *Journal of Adolescent Research, 10,* 427-448.

Paine-Andrews, A., Fawcett, S. B., Richter, K. P., Berkley, J. Y., Williams, E. L., and Lopez, C. M. (1996). Community coalitions to prevent adolescent substance abuse: The case of the "Project Freedom" replication initiative. *Journal of Prevention and Intervention in the Community, 14,* 81-99.

Rapoport, R. N. (1985). Research and action. In R. N. Rapoport (Ed.). *Children, youth and families: The action-research relationship.* New York: Cambridge University Press.

Rappaport, J. (1977). *Community psychology: Values, research, and action.* New York: Holt, Rinehart & Winston.

Rappaport, J. (1987). Terms of empowerment/exemplars of prevention: Toward a theory for community psychology. *American Journal of Community Psychology, 15,* 121-148.

Rappaport, J. (1990). Research methods and the empowerment social agenda. In P. Tolan, C. Keys, F. Chertok, & L. Jason (Eds.). *Researching community psychology: Issues of theory and methods.* Washington, D.C.: American Psychological Association.

Serrano-Garcia, I. (1990). Implementing research: Putting our values to work. In P. Tolan, C. Keys, F. Chertok, & L. Jason (Eds.). *Researching community psychology: Issues of theory and methods.* Washington, D.C.: American Psychological Association.

Small, S. A. (1996). Collaborative, community-based research on adolescents: Using research for community change. *Journal of Research on Adolescence, 6,* 9-22.

Zimmerman, M. A. & Rappaport, J. (1988). Citizen participation, perceived control, and psychological empowerment. *American Journal of Community Psychology, 16,* 725-750.

Zimmerman, M. A., Israel, B. S., Schulz, A., & Checkoway, B. (1992). Further explorations in empowerment theory: An empirical analysis of psychological empowerment. *American Journal of Community Psychology, 20,* 707-727.

Zimmerman, M. A. (in press). Empowerment theory: Psychological, organizational, and community levels of analysis. In J. Rappaport & E. Seidman (Eds.). *Handbook of community psychology.* New York: Plenum.

Ongoing Evaluation
in AIDS-Service Organizations:
Building Meaningful Evaluation Activities

Robin Lin Miller
University of Illinois at Chicago

J. Brian Cassel
Gay Men's Health Crisis, Inc.

SUMMARY. Expectations by foundations and federal, state, and city funders that *HIV-prevention* programs in *AIDS-service organizations* document their effectiveness have dramatically increased over the last decade. Unfortunately, current demands for outcome-oriented *program evaluation* have resulted in evaluations that do not produce useful information for program staff or for improving HIV prevention efforts in general. This paper argues that there are four main causes of substandard evaluation. A model for producing evaluation results that are useful and interpretable is proposed. *[Article copies available for a fee from The Haworth Document Delivery Service: 1-800-342-9678. E-mail address: getinfo@haworthpressinc.com <Website: http://www.haworthpressinc.com>]*

Address correspondence to: Robin Lin Miller, PhD, University of Illinois at Chicago, Department of Psychology (M/C 285), 1007 West Harrison Street, Chicago, IL 60607-7137.

The authors gratefully acknowledge the assistance of Doug Bell, Ron Stall, and Joseph P. Stokes for comments on the ideas expressed in this paper.

This paper is based on an invited address delivered by Robin Lin Miller at the 1995 National Gay and Lesbian Health Foundation Annual Conference.

[Haworth co-indexing entry note]: "Ongoing Evaluation in AIDS-Service Organizations: Building Meaningful Evaluation Activities." Miller, Robin Lin, and J. Brian Cassel. Co-published simultaneously in *Journal of Prevention & Intervention in the Community* (The Haworth Press, Inc.) Vol. 19, No. 1, 2000, pp. 21-39; and: *HIV/AIDS Prevention: Current Issues in Community Practice* (ed: Doreen D. Salina) The Haworth Press, Inc., 2000, pp. 21-39. Single or multiple copies of this article are available for a fee from The Haworth Document Delivery Service [1-800-342-9678, 9:00 a.m. - 5:00 p.m. (EST). E-mail address: getinfo@haworthpressinc.com].

KEYWORDS. HIV-prevention, AIDS-service organizations, program evaluation

As the number of HIV prevention programs and their cost have increased, so have expectations among program funders that the effectiveness of programs be demonstrated. Funders are demanding that organizations engage in increasingly sophisticated program evaluation activities. Although more programs are being evaluated, few evaluations have been conducted with sufficient skill and rigor to result in useful information. For example, to date only about three evaluations of community-based prevention programs have been published in peer-refereed journals, one indicator of research quality.

Although this phenomenon is not limited to HIV-prevention programs in community-based organizations, AIDS-service organizations are particularly in need of good evaluation. First, most AIDS-service organizations' financial survival is dependent upon maintaining positive relationships with a limited number of funders. Failure to demonstrate that funds are well spent in a particular program could lead to possible withdrawal of funds that could result in an agency's closure. Second, AIDS-service organizations are pioneers of creative responses to target populations that have been traditionally difficult to serve effectively in mainstream, public health programs. Documenting how AIDS-service organizations conceptualize and implement programs is critical to developing a body of knowledge about effective social programming for these underserved populations. It is also critical information if programs are to be replicated in other environments. Third, in an increasingly conservative political climate, HIV-prevention programs are especially vulnerable to defunding. Accusations that HIV-prevention programs "encourage" drug use, homosexuality, and promiscuity maintain currency in many political and social circles. Good evaluation can be an important tool for influencing policies to support HIV prevention efforts. Finally, good evaluation is a critical tool for improving the work of AIDS-service organizations.

Several factors have contributed to evaluations that do not provide useful, interpretable information.

Resources. This scenario is familiar to most AIDS-service organizations, and probably, to most community-based organizations:

Your organization has received a $50,000 foundation grant to start an innovative new program. The funding is to cover the salary of the program's coordinator and the nonpersonnel service costs of the program. A condition of the grant is that the program be evaluated for its effectiveness. However, only about $2,000 of the grant can be applied to the evaluation, after the program costs are accounted for. If you are to fulfill the funder's mandate, you will have to take money away from some other program in your organization to conduct the evaluation.

Setting aside the fact that it would be inappropriate to conduct an effectiveness evaluation of a program in its infancy, $2,000 is an entirely inadequate sum of money to conduct a good evaluation. An important cause of mediocre program evaluations is inadequate resources.

Funders frequently want organizations to conduct evaluations that the funder is unwilling to pay for (National Community AIDS Partnership, 1993). Running a good program costs money and so does conducting a useful evaluation. If funders want AIDS-service organizations to conduct good evaluations, funders must be willing to pay the costs of conducting the evaluations. Beyond the limited support provided by program funders, few initiatives have specifically supported evaluation efforts in AIDS-related community organizations. Two model initiatives, one launched by the Health Services Improvement Fund of New York City and the education programs of the American Foundation for AIDS Research, no longer provide evaluation funds to AIDS-related community-based organizations. Without financial support commensurate with the cost of conducting sound evaluations, it is likely that current demand for rigorous evaluations will continue to result in evaluations of low quality and limited usefulness.

Expertise. Few AIDS-service organizations have within them people who are skilled program evaluators whose job it is to evaluate the organization's programs (National Community AIDS Partnership, 1993). Indeed, of the estimated 18,000 AIDS-service organizations in North America (Altman, 1994), only one has a department of internal evaluation research and only a handful of other relatively large organizations have either a part-time staff person who conducts evaluation or an ongoing relationship with local evaluation experts. The task of conducting program evaluation activities often falls to a staff person without evaluation expertise, to a graduate student in need of data, or to a consultant who may or may not have any training in program evaluation. The unfortunate result is evaluations that neither answer the questions they are intended to address, nor contribute to our knowledge base about effective social programs. Additionally, when evaluations are conducted by persons with only modest exposure to evaluation research methods, the resulting studies are often inappropriate and poorly executed, characterized by unsound measures, improperly coded and analyzed data, unethical treatment of participants, and misinterpreted findings. Unfortunately, examples of poorly executed studies are widespread. AIDS prevention evaluations often require information about participants' sexual and drug-using behavior, sexual partners, and other information about sensitive aspects of individuals' lives. In several instances known to the authors, inexperienced evaluators failed to provide respondents with informed consent and adequate confidentiality protection. Not only are ethical problems common, but shoddy execution in these sensitive areas leads to data of questionable validity.

Whether evaluators are internal or external to an organization, they should know something about program evaluation, which is a distinct discipline. Far too often the people who are conducting evaluations in AIDS-service organizations are unfamiliar with it and have too many other job responsibilities to pay adequate attention to conducting evaluations.

Models of program evaluation. The notion of a program evaluation held by many people working in AIDS, including funders, is based on the model of a university-based intervention research demonstration project. The central question addressed by such studies is whether X intervention produces detectable, desired changes among a group of participants. Although the demonstration project model can be considered a special case of program evaluation, it does not reflect the scope of activities that fall under the rubric of program evaluation.

The scientific paradigm guiding the design of demonstration projects draws heavily on the classic, randomized experiment. Internal validity is of paramount concern. The researcher attempts to control all possible competing explanations for change in participants' behavior, in part by creating an environment that is low in realism. External validity is often low in these experiments (Cronbach, 1982) and interventions are reduced to "black boxes." In the experimental paradigm, nuances of program delivery and context are considered noise. In contrast, program evaluation is concerned with the intervention's impact on participants, but it is also concerned with systematically investigating all of the things that surround it, such as the adequacy of the space and the staffing, whether what is planned on paper is actually what happens, how internal politics and stakeholder interests affect buy-in to the program, whether the program has unintended positive and negative consequences, and whether individuals' needs are met (Rossi & Freeman, 1995; Shadish, Cook, & Leviton, 1991). Thus, where demonstration projects are most often narrowly concerned with understanding whether manipulations in X lead to changes in Y, program evaluation is concerned with if, how, when, where, and why the features of social programs and the interventions embedded within them lead to desired and undesired social change.

We would argue that for almost all AIDS-service organizations, the demonstration project model is inappropriate. Though evaluators debate the role of classic experiments in evaluation (Conrad, 1994), most recognize that effective randomization and classic experimentation is difficult to achieve in many service delivery settings, and may also be inappropriate and unethical. Staff may be opposed to withholding services from individuals in a comparison group and sabotage randomized experiments (Devine, Wright, & Joyner, 1994). Experimentation may alter the way in which services are delivered so much that studying how the program actually operates becomes impossible.

One purpose of a demonstration project is to establish whether a given intervention works before it is widely disseminated. This type of experiment is most appropriate to that particular stage in a program's evolution, and not as a way to monitor the ongoing effectiveness of it. Most organizations are funded to develop and implement a program rapidly and broadly, skipping the stage of program development in which a classic experiment might produce maximally useful information. Programs frequently move directly from the idea stage to full dissemination in a manner consistent with the organization's primary role as a service provider. Funders contribute to this pattern of quick movement to dissemination by funding programs for 1 or 2 years, but expecting that service units are delivered monthly across the life of the funding. Imposing a demonstration project model on a fully disseminated, ongoing program makes little sense. In addition, since AIDS-service organizations are not set up like the research institutes that are capable of performing demonstration projects, the demonstration project model imposes an unreasonable standard of evaluation performance on organizations.

Misapplying a demonstration project model to program evaluation can result in substandard evaluations by leading us to ask only a very limited set of questions about a program, by pushing us to ask outcome questions about programs that have not been completely developed or are so small that they are unlikely to have a detectable behavioral impact, and by encouraging us to treat as background noise the very thing we want to understand–the program.

Politics. Evaluation is a political enterprise, and politics can affect the rigor and usefulness of evaluations (Dial & Stevens, 1994). Sometimes a manager or program staff person does not want to ask pertinent questions in an evaluation, so the evaluators avoid asking questions that might lead to the program's improvement. Sometimes managers do not want evaluation findings known, leading to the suppression of results. Sometimes staff do not buy into the evaluation and sabotage it. Sometimes a funder insists on particular data being collected that have no useful purpose for the program's staff, so the data are collected without care and are not used. Sometimes evaluators have their own organizational agenda that is imposed on the evaluation.

Although the evaluation literature is replete with discussions of how to encourage utilization of evaluation data (see, for example, Finne, Levin, & Nilssen, 1995; Patton, 1986; Weiss, 1972, 1981; Wholey, 1977) and with strategies to avoid misuse of evaluation data, this literature has not been widely applied to thinking about evaluation in HIV. Unfamiliarity with the lessons learned about evaluation politics over the past 20 years is perhaps most apparent among AIDS-service organizations in the common practice of program staff acting as evaluators of their own programs. Although it is not necessarily the case that evaluating one's own program is automatically biasing, there has been little discussion of the pros and cons of this widespread practice and few efforts have been made to manage potential biases. Innovations in evaluation such as Wholey's evaluability assessment (Wholey, 1977), Patton's utilization-focused evaluation (Patton, 1986), and the recent growth of empowerment evaluation (Fetterman, Kaftarian, & Wandersman, 1996) have had little impact on the ways in which community-based evaluation in AIDS is practiced. Given the tendency to use program staff as evaluators, the ideas stemming from the evolving literature in evaluation practice are timely and informative, yet few of these ideas have had a significant impact on the way in which evaluation is practiced in community-based HIV-related efforts.

Inadequate resources, limited expertise, poor understanding of program evaluation, and inattention to evaluation politics are all key factors in how the current pressure for more evaluation has resulted in evaluations of limited merit. It is key that we develop a clearer conceptualization of program evaluation to address the downward trend in evaluation quality. It is also imperative that we decide what we want to learn from program evaluations in community-based organizations and how we want to use that information.

TOWARD A BETTER MODEL OF PROGRAM EVALUATION IN COMMUNITIES

In this section, we will review basic program evaluation activities, providing illustrative examples of work conducted by the Evaluation Research Department at Gay Men's Health Crisis (GMHC). Then we will describe the history and structure of the department, offering it as a model for promoting evaluation efforts in AIDS-related organizations.

A brief primer in program evaluation. According to Shadish and colleagues (Shadish, Cook, & Leviton, 1991), program evaluation is concerned with assessing how much a program or policy improves the welfare of some group or community, how it does so, and how it can do so more effectively. Program evaluation activities are generally broken down into several categories, which parallel the stages of developing a sound program. These categories are often broadly described as formative and summative. The distinction between the two was portrayed by Robert Stake who said, "When the cook tastes the soup, it's formative. When the guests taste the soup, it's summative."

The basis for good programs and for good outcome evaluations begins with needs assessment. Needs assessment answers questions such as "what is the scope and severity of the problem," "what mechanisms would produce change," "what does the target population need and want," and "how relevant is my program to the solution?" Many programs are based on the vaguest notions of need and few programs take seriously the notion that needs change over time. One of the ways we sought to improve programs at GMHC was to infuse need analyses into program and agency decision-making processes. For example, GMHC's research department has engaged in eliciting clients' needs using focus group and qualitative interview methodologies (GMHC, 1995a; GMHC, 1996a) with randomly selected client samples. One use of the data was to help GMHC develop a five-year strategic plan. In another case, we conducted focus groups, again with randomly selected client samples, to understand how clients manage treatment-related issues, including self-advocacy with physicians (GMHC, 1994a). One finding of these focus groups was that GMHC's current treatment education activities did not meet the needs of women and families as well as other clients. In other cases, needs assessments took the form of literature reviews (for example, GMHC, 1991), providing staff with current information on intervention strategies and target populations.

Formative evaluation attempts to answer a range of questions. One type of formative evaluation examines which of two or more alternatives works better. For example, one could test two versions of a brochure with target audience members before deciding which one to print. In assessing two versions of a brochure at GMHC, we found that the version intended for clients with lower-literacy skills was perceived by clients as patronizing and confusing, rather than as easy-to-read, whereas clients of all literacy levels found the high-literacy skills version clear and informative (GMHC, 1994b). Clients also found the initial design and layout of the brochures unattractive and difficult to read, particularly for those clients who had suffered visual impairment due to CMV retinitis. Other findings included that information that was important to parents was not discussed (e.g., how to prevent children from being exposed to tuberculosis), that some information was confusing, and that there were content discrepancies between the Spanish-language and English-language versions of the materials. The formative evaluation saved the agency several thousand dollars in printing and mailing costs, far more than what it cost us to do the evaluation. Follow-up research suggested that GMHC produced a brochure that has been well received by clients and the city's tuberculosis control unit staff (GMHC, 1995b).

Program implementation evaluation examines the extent to which programs' operations are consistent with the objectives and procedures devised for them. That is, if anything is happening at all, does what actually happens on a day-to-day basis reflect what is supposed to happen, and if not, why? Implementation evaluation is particularly important, because without it, one could end up evaluating a program that was never implemented (Patton, 1986). For example, we monitored many aspects of an agency-wide tuberculosis control program (GMHC, 1994c). The evaluation uncovered that some parts of a planned training did not actually happen. Had we simply examined whether the participants' had the desired skills at the end of the training, we would have concluded that what was designed did not work, rather than that it did not happen, and GMHC might have mistakenly discarded a good training. In a 4-year evaluation we examined the effect of policy changes in client intake to manage caseload growth (GMHC, 1993). Although intended to be a quickly implemented, short-term response to the problem of caseload management, we found that the policy did not go into effect for over 15 months and is still in effect over 4 years later. We also found that the policy did not have any impact on caseload growth and that it produced multiple, undesired negative consequences.

Process evaluation is perhaps the most common request by funders and is the type of evaluation that most organizations do to some extent. Process evaluation examines what services are actually being delivered and to whom. Process evaluation includes counting service units delivered, writing curricula, describing policies and procedures, assessing consumer satisfaction, and so on, but it also explicitly compares these kinds of data to a program's goals and objectives. For example, in the tuberculosis evaluation we monitored installation and use of HEPA filters relative to established goals for when and where the filters were to be installed and how often they were to be in use. From the evaluation data, we learned that these very expensive filters were so noisy that people turned them off frequently, defeating the purpose of having them (GMHC, 1994d). Because of the evaluation, we detected the problem very quickly after the equipment was installed and the data allowed the agency to devise procedures for reducing the noise and making sure that the filters were on. As another example, the tuberculosis training mentioned earlier was considered mandatory for all employees, and GMHC staff kept careful records of who signed in at the beginning of the training in order to monitor attendance. However, our observers noted that there was significant attrition among trainees throughout the day (GMHC, 1994c). Our observation data suggested that fewer individuals were actually trained than the sign in data suggested. In another evaluation, we conducted telephone interviews with a large, randomly selected group of clients regarding their satisfaction with the services that GMHC provides. While clients were generally satisfied with the services that they received, we identified several aspects of service provision that could be improved, such as keeping clients informed of the status of legal and advocacy cases, even if nothing had changed, and increasing client input into all programs (GMHC, 1994e).

It is a common tenet of program evaluation that all summative studies must also include at least some aspects of process evaluation in order to be valid, useful, and meaningful. Sometimes it is appropriate to conduct only the formative level of evaluation. Formative evaluation activities are essential to understand how programs can be improved and why they may or may not ultimately meet their objectives. In contrast, outcome evaluation answers questions such as "did the program make a difference?" and "if knowledge was supposed to increase, did it?" Outcome evaluation not only requires an examination of whether desired changes occurred, but also whether alternative explanations for any observed changes can be ruled out. The simple pretest-posttest design used so often in AIDS-service organizations cannot rule out most rival explanations for findings: people are only compared with themselves, and so observed changes could reflect natural change rather than change resulting from the intervention, simply completing a questionnaire could produce observed changes, other events that occurred at the same time as the program could produce observed changes, and so on (Campbell & Stanley, 1963, Cook & Campbell, 1979). The simple pretest-posttest design also lacks construct validity, primarily due to mono-operation bias and failure to select a representative sample of treatments (Cook & Campbell, 1979). The simple pretest-posttest design is most accurately viewed as a way to assess program processes and not program achievement (Peterson, Card, Eisen, & Sherman-Williams, 1994).

The job of a program evaluator–to develop adequate outcome evaluation designs that minimally disrupt service delivery and at the same time capture how the program really works–can be quite difficult. For example, we conducted a 2-year study of a GMHC safer sex workshop. We examined whether men who had attended the workshop reported increases in self-efficacy, positive condom attitudes, positive beliefs about safer sex, and condom use relative to their own pretest scores and to a comparison group of men who were equally motivated to change at 1 and 4 months after the workshop (Miller, 1994; Miller, 1995). We found that behavior did not change, although attitudes, beliefs, and self-efficacy did change. Since the program was theory-driven, we also assessed whether the program's theory was consistent with the data. The results suggested that the program's theory was consistent with the data, implying that the manipulations in the program might have been too weak to produce behavior change or that the self-selected group of men who attended this program had little room for behavioral improvement. Process data suggested that the program facilitators were not following the program curriculum rigorously and had made changes that would dilute the intervention's impact. Quantitative and interview data also suggested that the program was attracting a group of men who engaged in relatively low levels of risk behavior. The evaluation led to changes in the way facilitators were trained and monitored. The program was also redesigned to have a better chance of meeting its objectives.

Cost-effectiveness and cost-benefit evaluation compares program costs with expected benefits, or compares the cost differences of alternative program strategies. For example, one could study whether two different needle exchange programs have similar benefits, but different costs. While they are computationally easy studies to conduct, cost-oriented evaluations are particularly difficult to perform because what costs should be included and how to value them are difficult. What is the value of volunteer time? Should capital, indirect, and overhead costs be included in an estimate? How should costs that are not stable over time be estimated? The costs of providing meals to homebound people with AIDS depends on seasonal costs in ingredients and in the number of people who are fed day to day. At GMHC, our philosophy has been that too few programs have yet had the benefit of improvement-oriented evaluation activities for it to be appropriate to subject them to this type of study. For example, few programs have fully-documented curricula, or training and policies and procedures manuals. The quality of record-keeping systems varies widely among programs, as does consistency of implementation. Without basic program documentation, it would be difficult to know what we were evaluating. We believe that unless these basic forms of documentation are developed, program implementation is assessed, and implementation problems are corrected, sophisticated cost-effectiveness studies are premature.

Finally, impact evaluation answers the question "did the program make a difference?" Here the interest is in the program's ultimate impact, for example, reduced HIV seroconversion, rather than on more proximal attitudinal and behavioral outcomes such as intentions to reduce risk and increased condom use. For most AIDS-service organizations, impact evaluation would be nearly impossible to conduct, in part because many of the programs AIDS-service organizations provide are full coverage programs for a local area. In our view, the cost, complexity, and difficulty of conducting this type of study make it beyond the means of an AIDS-service organization.

Ideally, each of these types of evaluation form successive stages of program development. Realistically, not all organizations have the capacity to engage in all of these activities. However, most organizations have the capacity to engage in some of them, especially the process and formative tasks.

All organizations should be able to develop precise, up-to-date statements of the problem and target population that a particular program is designed to address. Stating the problem is essential to identify what the intervention can best address, what resources are necessary, and what conditions would indicate the problem had been solved (Peterson, Card, Eisen, & Sherman-Williams, 1994). All organizations should make explicit statements of goals and objectives for each of their programs. Goals and objectives are the basis for evaluating the program and should be measurable. Goals are broad statements of a program's intended impact. Objectives are measurable, but not necessarily quantified, statements of how goals are to be met. For example, a program's goal might be to increase the proportion of adult gay men living in Chelsea who use condoms by 10% within two years, and one of its objectives might be that 50% of program participants will consistently use condoms for one year. All organizations should describe the specific programmatic actions that are designed to meet the program's objectives, specifying how long the program will last, how much of the program a participant would need to be exposed to for change to occur, and so on. This is in part an exercise in stating the program's theory. Having a well documented program rationale and action plan are fundamental in assessing a program, and all organizations should develop this kind of basic documentation.

All organizations should keep track of program recipients, although the sophistication of tracking may vary. Knowing who is served, for example, or who drops out is essential information to manage the program and on which to build evaluation. Depending on the complexity of the program, assessing the program's implementation may not be feasible for all organizations. However, assessing discrepancies between program plans and actual implementation is a fundamental step in conducting evaluation, as well as an aspect of quality management, and organizations should try to do at least that much. For example, we have conducted several analyses of our client database. These data have indicated inequities in service utilization across programs and have suggested that some programs are less well utilized by certain demographic groups than is desired. For example, though women and men were enrolled in Buddy services in proportion to their overall representation in the client population, women received about 50 percent fewer hours of the service than men (GMHC, 1996b).

Organizations may lack the capacity and resources to engage in more sophisticated program assessment than the basic steps described above. In fact, a majority of AIDS-service organizations may not be able to do more than what we have just described without straining their resources. However, so many organizations have not taken enough of these fundamental steps, that there is plenty of work to be done to document community programs and to evaluate them before we could ever get to the notion of outcome evaluations. In the absence of well documented program rationales, action plans, and participant tracking, program implementation, process, and outcome evaluations cannot be meaningfully performed and are premature. We believe that it is a poor use of resources to submit a program to outcome evaluation, if these more basic evaluation activities have not been completed. In fact, we would argue that concentration on rigorous formative evaluation activities is more likely to produce an increase in effective prevention programs in AIDS-service organizations than outcome evaluations. We urge funders and organizations to focus evaluation efforts on formative evaluation activities.

Unfortunately, the current reality is that many programs are asked to engage in evaluation activities that are not consistent with the organizations' current level of evaluation capacity. Consider the clandestine needle exchange program, operated by one or two volunteers, or the grassroots outreach worker who distributes condoms to sex workers. What level of evaluation is appropriate to expect from AIDS-service organizations such as these?

According to Love (1991), organizations move through seven stages in developing internal evaluation capacity. At first, evaluation occurs ad hoc. A particular program may be subject to evaluation, but other programs are virtually undocumented. Organizations then move toward a commitment to more systematic evaluation, perhaps by designating a staff person to take on evaluation activities. Subsequently, the basic documentation of programs may begin to occur. Organizations then begin to conduct goal-oriented or process evaluations. From there, organizations progress to conduct outcome evaluation. At stage six, organizations engage in cost-benefit and cost-effectiveness evaluation. Finally, organizations evolve toward prospective evaluation. At this stage organizations use data to plan for the future, rather than simply assess the past. Few organizations actually progress much beyond the early stages of evaluation capacity, and few funders who support small AIDS-service organizations may know enough about program evaluation to judge an organization's evaluation capacity accurately (Council on Foundations, 1993). We would tentatively suggest that GMHC is the only AIDS-service organization that has moved toward these latter stages, and so we will describe how and why GMHC developed such evaluation capacity.

GMHC's internal evaluation department. The process by which GMHC has begun developing its evaluation capacity is similar to what Love described. Evaluators have been part of GMHC since the mid-1980s. Several prevention demonstration projects were housed at GMHC then, and the regular prevention staff began to want to include evaluation in the ongoing programs. Evaluators were hired on an ad hoc basis to work on particular projects. In 1989, three GMHC departments created full-time internal evaluation positions, one to study efforts to recruit and retain volunteers, one to study prevention programs, and one to study efforts to care for people living with AIDS. With more than 8,000 volunteers, 40,000 to 100,000 participants annually in a variety of prevention programs, and more than 5,000 people with AIDS as clients, these early evaluators could barely scratch the surface of the evaluation needs of the organization, so the staff in each of these departments was steadily expanded. GMHC made its biggest commitment to evaluation in 1993 when it consolidated the staff in these various departments into a single program evaluation department. This consolidation occurred so that there could be consistent quality of research across the agency, all programs had access to evaluation resources, evaluation activities could reflect the agency's priorities, and evaluators were not reporting to program managers. This last concern is critical. One condition that has lead to the misuse of evaluation findings in many internal evaluation departments is that the department reports to someone other than the agency head. To avoid this potential source of misuse, GMHC decided that the department would report to the executive director (Cassel, 1995). Since the 1993 consolidation, GMHC has furthered its commitment by revising its mission statement to include the role of program evaluation in guiding decisions.

GMHC made a substantial financial commitment to support evaluation activities in the organization. In 1995, the department employed nine full-time and two part-time evaluators, as well as an administrative staff, several consultant evaluators, and a corps of about 50 volunteers. The department is responsible for evaluating the activities of 18 service departments, which house more than 100 distinct programs. The department established a committee on human subjects and a science advisory committee, both composed of external researchers. These two committees provide the department with advice on ethical and scientific issues. The department has also engaged university-based social scientists as advisors on many projects in order to have expert assistance and enhance the credibility of the department. In exchange for outside advice, we have created student research assistantships for graduate students. We have also sponsored agency-wide monthly colloquia, so that researchers and agency staff have regular opportunities to share information and ideas.

Despite the healthy size of the department, its resources are inadequate for the enormity of its task. For example, in 1995 the department's annual budget was less than 4% of the amount of money devoted to services, rather than the 12% Love recommends. The department must frequently turn down requests from staff and managers because it does not have the money or personnel to take on projects.

The Evaluation Research Department's mission is to use social science research methods to help ensure that the highest possible quality of service is provided by GMHC to people living with HIV/AIDS and to all at risk of HIV infection. Although the long-term goals are to document the caliber of selected GMHC programs and help ensure that program resources are used wisely, the department's initial emphasis was to help ensure that programs served the needs of people who received GMHC services; to analyze the goals that were established for programs in prevention and client programs critically; and to help ensure programs had well-defined objectives, reached the targeted clients, and were adequately documented. The department's initial emphasis reflected the state of documentation of programs. Early projections were that it would take at least until 1998 before the department could conduct meaningful outcome evaluations on a routine basis. The department does have to conduct outcome evaluations on programs that are not, in the research staff's view, appropriate candidates for it, but staff try in those cases to advocate for extensive formative research activities to be included in the evaluation. Staff have also sought to structure several contracts so that the research department selected which program was adequately prepared for an outcome evaluation, rather than the funder.

The department also serves another critical function as the gatekeeper for external researchers who want to study GMHC's consumers or seek GMHC's endorsement of their research. In a single year, GMHC receives more than 50 requests to recruit research subjects via the agency and provide letters of support for grants. The department and its advisory committees make sure that GMHC receives adequate information to judge the merit of the research, that human subjects' issues have been attended to, and that the researchers are committed to inform GMHC of study results.

Although the growth of evaluation capacity at GMHC has taken many years, and its evolution remains incomplete, the benefits of the investment in simple evaluation activities have begun to emerge. New funders have been attracted by GMHC's capacity to document its efforts. Clients have had more voice in the way in which programs are delivered and view the agency as more responsive to their needs. Managers have better information about what is going on in the programs they oversee. Staff have had increased ability to detect problems early with minimal burden. Several costly errors have been averted because of early detection of problems in evaluation research activities. Technology transfer from behavioral science and intervention research occurs regularly. Evaluation data has also celebrated the organization's achievements and improved its functioning in multiple arenas. While the road to a productive collaboration has been rocky, our experience suggests that tailored, adequately-funded evaluation can improve an organization's functioning and contribute to knowledge about good social programming.

CONCLUSION

A seasoned evaluator once asked us, "Why are you people in AIDS prevention so anxious to have every tiny program demonstrate it is effective? We don't expect every physician to demonstrate that penicillin is effective each time it is prescribed, although we do expect someone has demonstrated it before physicians prescribe it widely. Isn't it more useful to know when, how, to whom, and why a physician makes a prescription and that she gives a prescription that matches the patient's condition?" While it was not the best analogy, it was a good question. At the heart of it, we believe that the AIDS-related community of service providers, funders and scientists need to decide what it is we want to know about ongoing AIDS prevention programs in AIDS-service organizations and whether we are willing to get the resources that are necessary to answer whatever those questions are. As we engage in that dialogue, we urge that the lessons we have learned about evaluating HIV prevention and service programs at GMHC be considered.

First, all programs are worthy of good documentation. You can not make good decisions about what to evaluate, what not to evaluate, and how programs can be improved, if the programs are not well described.

Second, formative evaluations can be good evaluations. We encourage organizations to conduct the best possible formative evaluations they can, rather than prematurely or inappropriately conducting poor outcome evaluations. We stand to learn more about how things really work by focusing on the formative. We will also avoid becoming co-conspirators in undermining the standards of good evaluation.

Third, not all programs merit outcome evaluation, and some merit only a little. Some programs are too small-scale to be likely to have a detectable effect. It is not a good use of resources to conduct an outcome evaluation when a detectable outcome is unlikely to occur. Rather, we should focus on good formative evaluation for such programs.

Fourth, if the findings of an excellent evaluation are not useful or utilized by an organization, it was not such an excellent evaluation after all. Utilization of findings to improve the work of community-based organizations is perhaps the most important goal for evaluators and program staff, once they have completed the data collection and analysis.

Fifth, it takes a long time and a lot of resources to build evaluation capacity in an organization. It is a worthwhile investment if you are serious about meeting your goals, but it is an investment that requires a long-term commitment, great patience, and resources.

REFERENCES

Altman, D. (1994). *Power and community: Organizational and cultural responses to AIDS*. Bristol, PA: Taylor & Francis.

Campbell, D. T., & Stanley, J. C. (1963). *Experimental and quasi-experimental designs for research*. Chicago, IL: Rand McNally.

Cassel, J. B. (1995, November). An internal evaluation of a controversial policy. Paper presented at the annual meeting of the American Evaluation Association, Vancouver, British Columbia.

Conrad, K. J. (Ed.). (1994). Critically Evaluating the Role of Experiments [special issue]. *New Directions in Program Evaluation, 63*, San Francisco, CA: Jossey-Bass.

Cook, T. D., & Campbell, D. T. (1979). *Quasi-experimentation: Design and analysis issues for field settings*. Chicago, IL: Rand McNally.

Council on Foundations. (1993). *Evaluation for foundations: Concepts, cases, guidelines, and resources*. San Francisco, CA: Jossey-Bass.

Cronbach, L. J. (1982). *Designing evaluations of education and social programs*. San Francisco, CA: Jossey-Bass.

Devine, J. A., Wright, J. D., & Joyner, L. M. (1994). Issues in implementing a randomized experiment in a field setting. In Conrad, K. J. (Ed.) Critically Evaluating the Role of Experiments [special issue]. *New Directions in Program Evaluation, 63*, (27-40). San Francisco, CA: Jossey-Bass.

Fetterman, D. M., Kaftarian, S. J., & Wandersman, A. (1996). *Empowerment evaluation: Knowledge and tools for self-assessment and accountability*. Newbury Park, CA: Sage.

Finne, H., Levin, M., & Nilssen, T. (1995). Trailing research: A model for useful program evaluation. *Evaluation, 1*(1), 11-31.

GMHC. (1991). *Double minorities: Black and Latino men who have sex with men*. New York, NY: GMHC.

GMHC. (1993). *Managing caseload growth in client services*. New York, NY: GMHC.

GMHC. (1994a). *Obtaining secondary prevention information and making health-related decisions*. New York, NY: GMHC.

GMHC. (1994b) . *Tuberculosis education and treatment support program, report 1*. New York, NY: GMHC.

GMHC. (1994c). *Tuberculosis education and treatment support program, report 2.* New York, NY: GMHC.

GMHC. (1994d). *Tuberculosis education and treatment support program, report 3.* New York, NY: GMHC.

GMHC. (1994e). *Client satisfaction survey.* New York, NY: GMHC.

GMHC. (1995a). *Clients' experiences and satisfaction with intake.* New York, NY: GMHC.

GMHC. (1995b). *Tuberculosis education and treatment support program, report 5.* New York, NY: GMHC.

GMHC. (1996a). *Assessing GMHC clients' needs.* New York, NY: GMHC.

GMHC. (1996b). *Patterns of service utilization in client programs.* New York, NY: GMHC.

Love, A. (1991). *Internal evaluation: Building organizations from within.* Newbury Park, CA: Sage.

Miller, R. L. (1994). *Safer sex maintenance among gay men.* Unpublished doctoral dissertation. New York: New York University.

Miller, R. L. (1995). Assisting gay men to maintain safer sex: An evaluation of an AIDS service organization's safer sex maintenance program. *AIDS Education and Prevention: An Interdisciplinary Journal, 7*(Suppl. 5), 48-63.

National Community AIDS Partnership. (1993). *Evaluating HIV/AIDS prevention programs in community-based organizations.* Washington, DC: Author.

Patton, M. (1986). *Utilization-focused evaluation.* Newbury Park, CA: Sage.

Peterson, J. L., Card, J. J., Eisen, M. B., & Sherman-Williams, B. (1994). Evaluating teenage pregnancy prevention and other social programs: Ten stages of assessment. *Family Planning Perspectives, 26*(3), 116-131.

Rossi, P. H., & Freeman, J. E. (1995). *Evaluation: A systematic approach,* 5th ed. Newbury Park, CA: Sage.

Shadish, W. R., Cook, T. D., & Leviton, L. C. (1991). *Foundations of program evaluation: Theories of practice.* Newbury Park, CA: Sage.

Stevens, C. J. & Dial, M. (Eds.). (1994). Preventing the Misuse of Evaluation [special issue]. *New Directions in Program Evaluation,* (64). San Francisco, CA: Jossey-Bass.

Weiss, C. H. (1972). *Evaluating action programs: Readings in social action and education.* Boston, MA: Allyn & Bacon.

Weiss. C. H. (1981) . Measuring the use of evaluation. In J. A. Ciarlo (Ed.), *Utilizing evaluation: Concepts and measuring techniques* (pp. 17-33). Newbury Park, CA: Sage.

Wholey, J. S. (1977). Evaluability assessment. In L. Rutman (Ed.), *Evaluation research methods: A basic guide.* Newbury Park, CA: Sage.

Influence of Health Beliefs, Attitudes and Concern About HIV/AIDS on Condom Use in College Women

Doreen D. Salina
Northwestern University

Lisa Razzano
University of Illinois at Chicago

Linda Lesondak
Georgia State University

SUMMARY. Acquired Immune Deficiency Syndrome (AIDS) represents a significant health risk for all sexually active adults. Women, in particular, may be at greater risk of HIV infection due to attitudes and beliefs which interfere with initiating and maintaining consistent condom usage. One hundred twenty-six college women completed a survey which measured the impact of sex role ascription, drug and alcohol use patterns, number of partners and sexual history in predicting condom usage. Additional factors explored include attitudes towards condoms, health beliefs, and present and future concern about contracting HIV/AIDS from a sexual partner. Findings indicate that intent to use condoms in the future was associated with greater present and future concern about contracting HIV/AIDS. In regression analyses, only

---

Address correspondence to: Doreen D. Salina, PhD, 401 North Michigan Avenue, Suite 1200, Chicago, IL 60611.

The authors would like to gratefully acknowledge Leonard Jason, PhD, Professor, Department of Psychology, DePaul University for his invaluable input and support of this work.

[Haworth co-indexing entry note]: "Influence of Health Beliefs, Attitudes and Concern About HIV/ AIDS on Condom Use in College Women." Salina, Doreen D., Lisa Razzano, and Linda Lesondak. Co-published simultaneously in *Journal of Prevention & Intervention in the Community* (The Haworth Press, Inc.) Vol. 19, No. 1, 2000, pp. 41-53; and: *HIV/AIDS Prevention: Current Issues in Community Practice* (ed: Doreen D. Salina) The Haworth Press, Inc., 2000, pp. 41-53. Single or multiple copies of this article are available for a fee from The Haworth Document Delivery Service [1-800-342-9678, 9:00 a.m. - 5:00 p.m. (EST). E-mail address: getinfo@haworthpressinc.com].

41

number of previous sexual partners was significantly related to condom use. *[Article copies available for a fee from The Haworth Document Delivery Service: 1-800-342-9678. E-mail address: getinfo@haworthpressinc.com <Website: http://www.haworthpressinc.com>]*

KEYWORDS. HIV/AIDS, sex-roles, HIV and condom use, women and AIDS

Acquired Immunodeficiency Syndrome (AIDS) presents a growing and significant health problem for women. In the United States alone, more than 70,000 women have been diagnosed with AIDS to date, and the disease has become one of the five leading causes of death in women of reproductive age in the United States. Unprotected heterosexual behavior continues to place women at risk for HIV transmission and is identified as the route responsible for infection in more than half of the women currently diagnosed with AIDS (CDC, 1997). Other than abstinence, consistent use of latex condoms is the only proven effective method of reducing the risk of HIV infection. Younger women in particular may be at greater risk because of developmental factors such as sexual experimentation with multiple partners, drug and alcohol use and a general belief that they are invulnerable.

Many young adults have never used condoms, and those who do report inconsistent use patterns (DiClemente, 1992). It has been well documented that despite college students' high level of knowledge regarding HIV/AIDS, knowledge level does not necessarily translate into behavior change related to condom usage. It is essential, therefore, that HIV/AIDS prevention programs address attitudes and behaviors associated with condom use with women and include them if these programs are to be effective.

There have been few studies which examine how women's attitudes towards their health directly relate to HIV/AIDS risk behavior and subsequent condom use. Women face additional challenges to practicing safer sex behaviors due to gender issues. Generally, because of cultural and social influences, women are considered less likely to initiate condom usage in intimate relationships due to differences in perceived or actual power within their intimate relationships (Campbell, Peplau, & DeBro, 1992). Sex role expectations have largely been ignored in HIV prevention programs (Salina, Hamilton & Leake,

1996) but may function as an additional barrier to a woman's ability to initiate and maintain consistent condom use with her sexual partner. Women who do insist that their partners use condoms risk rejection and accusations of unfaithfulness. Fear of negative consequences such as these may decrease the likelihood that women will attempt these types of safer sex negotiations and instead avoid potential conflict with their sexual partners through engaging in unprotected sexual behaviors. This failure to use condoms during all sexual encounters places women at relatively greater risk for HIV infection since HIV is more likely to be transmitted from men to women than from women to men, with some estimates of risk reaching seven to ten times more likely (Gath, 1992). In addition, since the overwhelming majority of people diagnosed with AIDS are men, one can assume that this pattern is also true for those infected with HIV but asymptomatic. This places women at greater probable odds of encountering an infected male sex partner (Peterson, Cates, & Curran, 1988).

The reasons why women report using condoms may be influential in understanding under what circumstances women use condoms. It may be that when women have concerns about HIV transmission, they may be more likely to consistently use condoms than when they believe they are not at risk. In addition, while some women may erroneously believe they are not at risk for HIV infection through unprotected sex, they may use condoms as a prevention for unwanted pregnancy since women remain primarily responsible for avoiding conception. If consistent use of condoms as a pregnancy prevention is occurring within a subset of women, it has the secondary value of reducing the risk of HIV transmission in women who may not be concerned with HIV. This phenomenon is germane to the context in which consistent condom use is promoted. For younger women who may not perceive themselves at risk for HIV, unwanted pregnancy may be more salient than risk of HIV/AIDS.

Attitudes towards women's specific sex roles within society and within relationships can impact on many aspects of safer sex behavior. Women who ascribe to more traditional beliefs about women may be less likely to engage in risk reduction behaviors. The extent to which women subscribe to traditional views may hamper HIV/AIDS prevention efforts and place women at greater risk of contracting HIV because of the perceived inappropriateness of either initiating safer sex negotiations or insisting on condom usage. A series of studies related to beliefs about what may be considered traditionally appropriate sex role behaviors of men and women has led to the construct of sex role Egalitarianism (Beere, King, Beere, & King, 1983; King & King, 1983a; 1983b). Egalitarianism can been described as holding attitudes that support nontraditional sex roles for both genders. Since traditionally men have been expected to decide on and provide for condom use, women who hold egalitarian attitudes may be more likely to accept responsibility for this task than women who ascribe to more traditional attitudes.

Other attitudes may be influential regarding condom use. The Health Belief Model has been used extensively to examine attitudes towards one's own health maintenance that are associated with life-style behaviors (Becker, 1974; Janz & Becker, 1984). The model postulates five dimensions associated in whether an individual chooses to utilize health protective behaviors. These include: (1) Perceived Susceptibility to the disease; (2) Perceived Self-Efficacy or the belief that one is capable of changing risk behaviors to avoid the disease; (3) Severity of the consequences of the disease; (4) Benefits of changing risk behaviors; (5) Barriers to carrying out these changes. More recently, researchers have attempted to apply the model to HIV/AIDS risk reduction. While the Health Belief Model has both strengths and limitations with respect to understanding HIV risk behavior, this conceptualization may be useful in understanding why some individuals continue to engage in risk behaviors despite generally high levels of knowledge about HIV. Mary Anne Hoffman (1992; 1994) created the Health Belief Model for AIDS Questionnaire by altering the HBM based on factor analytic studies with both men and women. According to these data, the responses for the self efficacy and barriers factors were better accounted for by combining these items into one factor which she called Distancing. Distancing refers to the respondent's belief that HIV is related to environmental factors outside of the control of the individual. Among other results, Hoffman found that higher frequency of condom use was associated with the self efficacy/barrier factor and with Perceived Susceptibility.

Attitudes towards condoms is another important factor that influences consistent condom use patterns. Campbell, Peplau, and De-Bro (1992) developed the Condom Attitude Scale to address the importance of four classes of attitudes as an index of the likelihood of using condoms. These four domains are: Comfort and Convenience; Efficacy as a method of both birth control and prevention of sexually transmitted diseases (STDs); Interpersonal concerns; and Sexual Sensation. The scale also includes a single item measure of general condom attitudes. Predicting future condom use for women was related to scores on the Interpersonal domain, the number of previous sex partners, the single item general attitude towards condoms and amount of concern expressed about contracting an STD (Campbell, Peplau & DeBro, 1992).

It is essential to identify which attitudes and beliefs are related to HIV protective behaviors and which are predictive of consistent condom usage in order to create more efficacious HIV/AIDS interventions. To this extent, we examined whether attitudes towards women's sex roles, level of concern about contracting HIV and number of sexual partners were influential in predicting condom use. We also examined whether health beliefs are effective in predicting current condom use in college aged women.

METHODS

Participants

One hundred twenty-six women volunteers were recruited from a private, urban midwestern university's Introduction to Psychology course. Sixty-seven percent of the women were Caucasian, 13% were Latina, 9% were Asian, 8% were African American, and 2% classified themselves as members of other racial/ethnic groups. Women's ages ranged from 17 to 37 years old, with a mean age of approximately 20 years old. All but four of the participants (97%) reported that they were heterosexual. Three women considered themselves bisexual, and one respondent identified as lesbian. Forty-four percent of the women reported that they knew a gay male, but only 18% indicated that they knew a lesbian.

Measures

Participants were asked to complete a series of questionnaires examining issues related to intimate relationships. These measures included demographic information, a comprehensive history regarding sexual activity, alcohol, and drug use, and the Crowne-Marlowe Social Desirability Scale (1964). None of the women in this sample received a score on the Crowne-Marlowe which placed them outside of the normative distribution, suggesting minimal or no attempt by the women to present themselves in a socially desirable and/or more favorable fashion. In addition, the questionnaires included the Condom Attitude Scale (CAS) (Campbell, Peplau, & DeBro, 1992), the Marital and Social-Interpersonal-Heterosexual subscales of the Sex Role Egalitarianism Scale (SRES) (King & King, 1983), and the Health Beliefs Model for AIDS Questionnaire (HBMQ) (Hoffman, 1992). The SRES consists of five scales, of which two were utilized for this project, the marital roles and the social-interpersonal heterosexual scale. These two scales contain items closely related to condom use and sexual behavior. The remaining scales, examining employment, parenting, and education were not included. Based on the reliability and validity data, it is possible to use them as separate measures. Included in the HBMQ are five subscales which examine: (1) distance; (2) severity; (3) self-efficacy; (4) susceptibility; and (5) benefits. Each of these paper-and-pencil measures as well as the identified subscales has stable realizability and validity coefficients (i.e., exceeding .60). Self-reported condom use was measured using a five-point Likert type scale ranging from 1 ("don't think about using one") to 5 ("always uses one"). The surveys also collected data on previous sexual and drug use behaviors, as well as asking the respondent to rate their present and future concern about contracting HIV. Future intentions to use a condom was assessed on a five point scale.

Procedure

Women reported to a laboratory and were administered the survey instruments in groups of approximately 15 students by two female experimenters. After obtaining signed informed consent, the experimenters instructed the participants that the purpose of the present research was to learn more about women's attitudes and concerns about health and intimate relationships. Participants also were informed that all of the material contained in their survey responses was anonymous and would be kept private and confidential. Once respondents had completed the survey, they were appropriately debriefed and any questions regarding the survey as well as the purposes of the research were addressed. Participants also were provided with information about HIV/AIDS prevention.

RESULTS

Data analyses first examined the zero-order relationships among the demographic, sex and drug history, and questionnaire sub- and total scales with Pearson correlations. These comparisons included, but were not limited to, relationships between outcomes such as condom use patterns, present and future concern regarding HIV infection, and future intention to use condoms, and variables related to past sexual behavior, use of birth control, and alcohol and drug use patterns. Once these relationships were explored, the information was used in order to develop and test the predictive relationships among these variables using regression analysis.

Use of Condoms, Other Birth Control Methods, and Previous Number of Partners

Of the 126 women in this sample, 35 (28%) reported never having sexual intercourse. Of the remaining 91 (72%) women, eight did not use any form of birth control, including condoms. Since the outcome is based on attitudes towards health and condoms, all of the women were included in subsequent analyses to allow examination of specific attitudes toward condom use. Data regarding condom use were collected by asking both how consistently the respondent used condoms on a five point scale and as part of collecting information about patterns of birth control. Data regarding birth control were examined in order to determine whether condoms were chosen more often than other methods. Examining women's responses regarding different methods of forms of birth control, among women who reported use of *any* method, 46% reported that they used condoms, 22% used the birth control pill, and 15% reported using the withdrawal method. Interestingly, among this sample, none of the respondents reported use of other barrier methods such as diaphragms or sponges. With regard to respondents' primary method of birth control, 58% reported choosing condoms, while only 23% reportedly chose the birth control pill. The number of women who identified withdrawal as their primary method was about 7%. In addition, data indicate that among women who reported any condom use, 39% of the respondents described consistent use (100% of the time), 53% used them occasionally or regularly (50-75%), while 8% infrequently (≤ 25%) used condoms. Of this sample, 34% reported having only one partner, 41% indicated two or three partners, while the remaining 25% reported four or more partners. The median number of partners reported by women in this sample was two.

Relationships Between Concern About HIV/AIDS, Health Beliefs, and Condom Use

Pearson correlations were used in order to examine the relationships among condom use patterns, present and future concern over HIV infection, and future intent to use condoms as a method of protection from HIV/AIDS. Several noteworthy significant relationships were revealed in these comparisons. For example, among the reasons noted for use of condoms, women noted prevention of unwanted pregnancy as well as prevention of STDs in general. Additionally, women reported that they were more likely to use condoms to reduce their risk for HIV infection. In fact, the greater level of present concern regarding HIV infection reported by the respondent, the more likely she was to report using condoms ($r = .29, p < .001$). In addition, a comparison was made between women's present concern about HIV and their perceived susceptibility based upon their behaviors, as measured by the Susceptibility subscale of the HBMQ. This analysis indicated a weak but significant relationship between these outcomes, such that women with greater concern about contracting HIV believed that they were engaging in health behaviors which made them less vulnerable to infection ($r = -.12, p < .05$). A significant relationship also was identified between present condom use patterns and future concern about HIV infection and intention to use condoms. Specifically, higher levels of present concern reflected higher levels of perceived future concern ($r = .28, p < .01$) as well as future intention to use condoms ($r = .24, p < .02$). Perceived future concern also was related to intention to include condoms at future sexual encounters ($r = .35, p < .001$). Significant relationships also were noted between number of sexual partners and present concern about HIV infection ($r = .22, p < .01$), and increased use of drugs ($r = .51, p < .001$)

and alcohol (r = .45, *p* < .001) before sex. Finally, relationships among the CAS, the HBMQ and the SRES were explored. Correlational analyses of these scales identified a significant relationship between health beliefs and condom attitudes such that more positive health beliefs (i.e., higher total HBMQ scores) were significantly related to more positive attitudes toward condoms (r = .28, *p* < .01). No significant relationships were identified between either the CAS or the two SRES subscales. In this sample, women reported extremely skewed attitudes on both the CAS and the SRES subscales. In general, women in this sample had extremely positive attitudes towards condoms and tended to rate themselves as strongly egalitarian in their attitudes towards appropriate sex role behavior.

Predicting Condom Use

A series of regression models were developed to examine what impact specific attitudes and beliefs have on consistent condom use as well as the impact of several other predictor variables (i.e., number of sexual partners, and use of drugs or alcohol before having sex). Models which examined total scores on the CAS and the HBMQ with the other predictor variables indicated no significant relationship to consistent condom use.

A subsequent regression model which examined the subscales of both the CAS and HBMQ was tested with the other predictor variables. This model is summarized in Table 1.

Interestingly, while none of the subscale measures were significantly related to condom use, number of previous partners was significantly related to the outcome. Furthermore, neither use of drugs nor alcohol before sex was significantly related to condom use.

The impact of egalitarianism on condom use also was tested. One model included the total Condom Attitude Scale as well as the combined egalitarianism measures (i.e., SRES social-interpersonal-heterosexual and marital subscales). Although this model was significant (F(5, 109) = 5.4, *p* < .001) and accounted for approximately 20% of the variance, the findings were similar to those described above. Specifically, only number of sexual partners significantly predicted condom use (*p* < .001). Finally, the subscales of the CAS and the SRES were entered into the model separately. While this regression analysis (summarized in Table 2) increased the amount of variance accounted for, the only predictor still significantly related to the outcome was number of sexual partners.

DISCUSSION

The results presented in this paper examined a subset of beliefs, attitudes and behaviors which may impact on consistent condom usage in a sample of college aged women. In general, women with more positive health beliefs were more likely to hold more positive attitudes towards condoms. This association did not translate into consistent condom usage, however, indicating that the role between attitudes and behaviors is mediated by other factors. In this sample, factors such as present and future level of concern about contracting HIV and multiple reasons given for condom use proved important. That women use condoms is apparent by the fact that almost 58% of the women in our sample who use birth control report that condom usage is their primary method. However, this usage is not universal, nor are these women reporting prophylactic use with each sexual encounter. Only 30% of the women reported using condoms all the time, leaving a significant number of sexually active women potentially at risk for exposure to HIV. The reasons respondents identified

TABLE 1. Summary of Regression Model Predicting Condom Use with Health Beliefs and Condom Attitudes

Variables in the Equation

Variable	B	SE B	Beta	T	Sig. T
Number of Partners	.156	.037	.445	4.16	.001***
HBMQ–Severity	−.008	.034	−.024	−.25	.804
HBMQ–Distance	.014	.016	.081	.85	.395
HBMQ–Benefits	−.005	.014	−.032	−.33	.739
HBMQ–Susceptibility	−.005	.014	−.033	−.33	.740
HBMQ–Barriers	−.005	.017	−.031	−.29	.770
CAS–Interpersonal	.033	.032	.098	1.03	.310
CAS–Efficacy	−.058	.039	−.137	−1.48	.141
CAS–Sexual	.043	.032	.122	1.33	.185
CAS–Communication	.002	.019	.012	.13	.898
Uses Drugs Before Sex	.157	.112	.141	1.40	.164
Uses Alcohol Before Sex	−.017	.074	−.025	−.23	.818
(Constant)	−.882	.995		−.88	.378

$R^2 = .25, F(12,103) = 2.83, p < .01$

using condoms were threefold: to avoid pregnancy, prevent sexually transmitted diseases in general and specifically to prevent HIV infection. This finding suggests that some women may use condoms consistently without regard to their HIV disease prophylactic abilities. This finding is important as it broadens the scope of HIV prevention efforts to include specific interventions within more general health promotion or pregnancy prevention programs. Women who might underestimate their own risk of contracting HIV but who use condoms as a birth control method are reducing their risk of HIV as well during times of use, but may unwittingly place themselves at risk through their failure to use condoms when not preventing pregnancy.

Condom use was also correlated with the amount of concern women expressed about contracting HIV with both present and future partners. In addition, actual condom use was predicted by the number of partners in this sample such that women with more sexual partners were actually using condoms more consistently. It may be that women with only one partner experience less concern about HIV infection because of a belief that their relationship is sexually monogamous. These women likely do not use condoms as much for HIV protection, but rather to avoid the complication of unwanted pregnancy. The women with more numerous partners reported more consistent condom use and may be more accurately identifying the potential for HIV infection as noted by their more elevated levels of both present and future concern.

TABLE 2. Summary of Regression Model Predicting Condom Use with Egalitarianism and Condom Attitudes

Variables in the Equation

Variable	B	SE B	Beta	T	Sig. T
Number of Partners	.162	.036	.460	4.47	.001***
SRES–Marital	.006	.009	.067	.68	.495
SRES–Soc.–Int.–Het.	−.006	.010	−.056	−.59	.565
CAS–Interpersonal	.025	.030	.073	.82	.416
CAS–Efficacy	−.061	.038	−.141	−1.59	.115
CAS–Sexual	.025	.029	.076	.87	.387
CAS–Communication	.0001	.019	.0009	−.01	.992
Uses Drugs Before Sex	.162	.111	.147	1.46	.146
Uses Alcohol Before Sex	−.027	.068	−.039	−.39	.696
(Constant)	−.519	.996		−.52	.604

$R^2 = .23$, $F(9, 105) = 3.48$, $p < .001$

The patterns of women's condom use will be strongly impacted by the reasons for use. Attitudes as well as specific behaviors such as number of sexual partners likely play a role in the decision whether and when to use condoms and should be explored in more depth in future research in women's sexual behavior. Additional studies need to identify which variables are important in predicting condom usage, and which attitudes are open to change which will facilitate consistent safer sex negotiations and behaviors. Our results suggest that women use condoms for a multitude of reasons and these findings should be incorporated in all health and pregnancy prevention programs as well as specific HIV/AIDS interventions.

REFERENCES

Baldwin, J. D., & Baldwin, J. I. (1988). Factors affecting sexual risk-taking behavior among college students. *Journal of Sex Research, 25*, 181-186.

Becker, M. H. (Ed.) (1974). The Health Belief Model and Personal Health Behavior. *Health Education Monographs, 2*, 324-473.

Bem, S. L. (1974). The measurement of psychological androgyny. *Journal of Consulting and Clinical Psychology, 42* (2), 155-162.

Beere, C. A., King, D. W., Beere, D. B., & King, L. A. (1983). The sex role egalitarianism scale: A measure of attitudes of equality between the sexes. *Sex Roles, 10*, 563-576.

Bouton, R. A., Gallaher, P. E., Garlinghouse, P. A., Leal, T., Rosenstein, L. D., & Young, R. K. (1987). Scales for measuring fear of AIDS and homophobia. *Journal of Personality Assessment, 51*(4), 606-614.

Campbell, S. M., Peplau, L. A., & Debro, S. C. (1992). Women, men and condoms: Attitudes and experiences of heterosexual college students. *Psychology of Women Quarterly, 16*, 273-288.

Catania, J. A., Dolcini, M. M., Coates, T. J., Kegeles, S. M., Greenblatt, R. M., & Puckett, S. (1989). Predictors of condom use and multiple partnered sex among sexually active women: Implications for AIDS-related health interventions. *Journal of Sex Research, 26*, 514-524.

Center for Disease Control. (1997, June). *HIV/AIDS Surveillance Report.* Atlanta, GA: CDC.

Chu, S. Y., Buehler, J. W., & Berkelman, R. L. (1990). Impact of the human immunodeficiency virus epidemic on mortality in women of reproductive age, United States. *JAMA, 264*, 225-229.

Crowne, D., & Marlowe, D. (1964). Social Desirability Scale, in *The Approval Motive.* New York: Wiley & Sons, Inc.

DiClemente, R. J. (1992). Psychosocial determinants of condom use among adolescents. In R. J. DiClemente (Ed.), *Adolescents and AIDS: A Generation in Jeopardy.* Newbury Park, CA: Sage Publications, Inc.

Gath, L. (1992, June). HIV and AIDS: Hitting hard at women. In *Positively Aware: The Monthly Journal of the Test Positive Aware Network*, 22-23.

Hoffman, M. A. (1992, August). *Development of the health belief model for AIDS questionnaire.* Paper presented at the annual convention of the American Psychological Association, Washington, D.C.

Janz, N. K., & Becker, M. H. (1984). The health belief model: A decade later. *Health Education Quarterly, 11,* 1-47.

King, D. W. & King, L. A. (1983). Sex-role egalitarianism as a moderator variable in decision-making: Two validity studies. *Educational and Psychological Measurement, 43,* 1199-1210.

Lee, H. (1989). Genital infection in female and male college students. *Journal of American College Health, 37,* 288-291.

Salina, D. D., Hamilton, A., & Leake, C. (1996). HIV and women. In I. Crawford and B. Fishman (Eds.). *Psychosocial Interventions in HIV Disease.* Northvale, New Jersey: Aronson, Inc.

Psychological Distress Among HIV-Impacted African-American and Latino Males

Rocco Domanico

Cook County Hospital, Chicago, Illinois

Isiaah Crawford

Loyola University, Chicago

SUMMARY. HIV infection is disproportionately more common among ethnic/racial minorities in the U. S., yet little research has examined how this population copes with their chronic illness. The available studies have primarily focused on white, middle class gay males. Little is known about the specific psychological responses and specific coping strategies of men from communities of color. While all people infected with HIV must cope with significant psychosocial stressors such as social stigmatization, and coping with a chronic and terminal illness, people of color likely face additional stressors related to homophobia and racism. This article presents a study of 100 men, 92% of which are men of color. Participants were recruited from a midwestern medical center and data were collected regarding the presence of psychological distress, coping styles, spirituality and sexual orientation. A series of analyses examined the relationship between these variables and specific coping methods. Results included a strong relationship be-

Address correspondence to: Isiaah Crawford, PhD, Chair, Department of Psychology, Loyola University, 6525 North Sheridon Road, Chicago, IL 60626.

[Haworth co-indexing entry note]: "Psychological Distress Among HIV Impacted African-American and Latino Males." Domanico, Rocco, and Isiaah Crawford. Co-published simultaneously in *Journal of Prevention & Intervention in the Community* (The Haworth Press, Inc.) Vol. 19, No. 1, 2000, pp. 55-78; and: *HIV/AIDS Prevention: Current Issues in Community Practice* (ed: Doreen D. Salina) The Haworth Press, Inc., 2000, pp. 55-78. Single or multiple copies of this article are available for a fee from The Haworth Document Delivery Service [1-800-342-9678, 9:00 a.m. - 5:00 p.m. (EST). E-mail address: getinfo@haworthpressinc.com].

tween increased positive mood when participants used an active coping style as compared with a passive-avoidant coping style. Greater levels of spiritual well being were correlated with positive mood. This article presents information on the psychological experience of ethnic/racial minority men who are HIV positive, have different coping styles and examines the role spirituality has in managing one's illness. *[Article copies available for a fee from The Haworth Document Delivery Service: 1-800-342-9678. E-mail address: getinfo@haworthpressinc.com <Website: http://www.haworthpressinc.com>]*

KEYWORDS. HIV infection, coping with HIV, spirituality and HIV

Since the discovery of the human immunodeficiency virus (HIV) and its etiological basis for Acquired Immune Deficiency Syndrome (AIDS) in 1983, a vast amount of research has been conducted to identify effective methods of prevention and treatment of its clinical syndromes. Research examining how individuals impacted by HIV emotionally contend with their illnesses has just recently been the target of specific investigation. Much of this research has addressed the experiences of middle-class, Caucasian, gay men. Very few studies have examined the psychological responses and coping strategies of ethnic/racial minority individuals impacted by HIV, although they account for 47% of individuals diagnosed with AIDS in the United States (CDC, 1996). The impact of psychosocial stressors such as social stigmatization, rejection, alienation, loss of employment and housing, and increased dependence on others associated with living with HIV has not been addressed adequately. Since there is evidence that chronic psychosocial stress seems to place HIV infected individuals at increased risk for experiencing opportunistic infections and other AIDS-related symptom exacerbation (i.e., Antoni, LaPerrier, Schneiderman, & Fletcher, 1989; Levy & Heiden, 1991; Schlesinger & Yodfat, 1989), methods of coping and adapting to these stressors may be important mediating variables to examine.

PSYCHOLOGICAL CORRELATES OF HIV INFECTION

Results from several studies indicate that anxiety, depression, and anger are the most common psychological correlates of HIV infection;

however, most individuals with HIV infection do not become chronically psychologically impaired (Burack, Barrett, & Stall, 1993; Faulstich, 1987; Kim, & Rickman, 1988; King, 1989; Markowitz, Rabkin, & Perry, 1994; and Siegal & Krauss, 1991). In his survey of 192 clients with HIV infection at two London hospital based clinics, King (1989) found that approximately 69% of the individuals did not evidence psychological impairment. Of the individuals presenting with psychological symptoms (31%), half experienced the onset of these problems following awareness of their HIV infection. This strongly suggests that some variable related to having HIV infection is associated with the onset or recurrence of psychopathology.

SPIRITUALITY AND COPING STRATEGIES

One potential method of intervention to decrease psychosocial distress is to develop or reinforce adaptive coping strategies in clients with HIV. There are numerous ways of initiating or strengthening existing coping strategies including increasing social networks, emphasizing spirituality, and/or altering deleterious behavioral or cognitive patterns (Gluhoski, 1996). Carson, Soeken, Shandy, and Terry (1990) address the importance of confronting the existential aspects of one's life, and discuss the impact of finding meaning in life and affirming a value in continuing to live.

Finding answers that fulfill these existential or spiritual questions has been found to lead to increased thoughts of hope, decreased negative affect, and a desire to live life to its fullest (Taylor, 1983). In fact, many people with AIDS (PWAs) are cognizant of the importance of hope, spirituality, and existential issues in coping with an HIV positive status. A majority of individuals with AIDS in the Carson et al. (1990) study linked their well-being to their own ability to reflect upon and derive answers regarding the existential and religious aspects of their lives. In comparing PWAs to individuals with HIV infection (i.e., non-AIDS), these researchers discovered that spirituality was directly associated with feelings of hope. Individuals were considered more hopeful if they had future expectations and positive thoughts about the future.

Another finding of interest in the Carson et al. (1990) study is that individuals with an AIDS diagnosis possessed significantly greater levels of hope than did HIV infected individuals despite the lack of difference between the two groups on factors of overall spiritual well-being. This is an interesting finding given that individuals with AIDS are further along in disease progression and can be expected to have more symptoms than are individuals who are HIV+ without AIDS. The authors report that these people with AIDS were usually long term survivors and they believed their well-being was linked to their ability to confront the existential questions that having AIDS elicits. The authors posit that feelings of being a survivor may serve to increase feelings of hope for PWAs. Consequently, assisting HIV infected individuals in their ability to find meaning in their lives and to develop adaptive coping strategies may reduce psychological distress and prolong periods of good health.

Namir, Wolcott, Fawzy, and Alumbaugh (1987) assessed the relationship among coping strategies, psychological variables, and physical well-being among 50 individuals diagnosed with AIDS. In their research, Namir and her colleagues identified three types of coping methods: active-cognitive; active-behavioral; and avoidance. An active-cognitive coping style is characterized by an appraisal of the stressful components of the illness and includes one's beliefs, attitudes, and thoughts about the illness. An active-behavioral coping strategy entails addressing specific problems as they arise and seeking out emotional, informational, and instrumental support from others when necessary. And finally, an avoidance coping approach involves attempting to evade or deny the reality of the illness by not attending to one's treatment protocol or self-medicating with alcohol or drugs (Namir et al., 1987). Using this system of categorizing coping behaviors, Namir et al. found in their sample of persons with AIDS those individuals who tended to utilize an avoidance coping strategy were more likely to feel depressed and to possess lower levels of self-esteem than their counterparts who managed the stressors of their illness by using active-behavioral coping strategies.

Capitaine, Szapocznik, Blaney, Morgan, Millon, and Eisdorfer (1990) examined whether ethnic/racial status, sexual orientation, and method of contracting HIV impacted on levels of perceived stress and the utilization of various coping strategies and behaviors of HIV infected Latino and Caucasian males. Their results indicated that Latino males experienced greater levels of daily stress than their Caucasian counterparts and that individuals who identified themselves as gay were more likely to utilize an avoidance and distancing coping style than their HIV impacted heterosexual peers (Capitaine et al. 1990). The authors attributed these findings to the increased prevalence of overt homophobic beliefs in Latino culture and the increased burden of concealing their sexual orientation for fear of experiencing additional social isolation and familial rejection. Capitaine and her colleagues also discovered that avoidance and distancing coping styles were the primary methods of coping among the HIV positive individuals in their study who were homosexual. These researchers posit that this is likely related to the additional stressors of social stigma, rejection, and alienation associated with being homosexual in a predominantly heterosexual society that generally does not condone homosexuality (Capitaine et al., 1990).

Additionally, Capitaine et al. (1990) point out that disclosing one's homosexuality to family and friends at the same time of disclosing one's HIV status is inherently stressful; consequently, individuals with a history of homosexual relationships/activities and a diagnosis of HIV who have not disclosed their sexual orientation with their social supports are likely to engage in more avoidant and distancing coping behaviors as a means of avoiding social rejection and alienation from their familial or community (i.e., ethnic/racial) support systems. This may account for the recent findings that indicate that African-American gay and bisexual men impacted by HIV are least likely to seek help from family members (Peterson, Coates, Catania, Hilliard, Middleton, & Hearst, 1995). The Capitone et al. (1990) findings are also consistent with Hays, Catania, McKusick, and Coates (1990) who found in their study, examining the impact of social support on the functioning of 530 gay men, that perceiving one's primary support system as being helpful and accessible was associated with lower levels of depression and anxiety.

Collectively, this research suggests that HIV impacted, gay-identified minority males may be at particular risk for experiencing psychological distress (i.e., stress) as a result of utilizing an avoidant coping strategy to contend with the social stigma and emotional sequelae associated with HIV and homosexuality in their communities. This avoidance of support networks may further compromise their immune systems and negatively impact their health status. This study is designed to examine some of these suppositions; specifically, the following hypotheses were developed: (1) HIV infected men who primarily utilize active-behavioral coping methods will be less psychologically distressed than their counterparts who predominately use avoidance coping methods; (2) gay and bisexual men of color with HIV will report more psychological distress than their heterosexual counterparts; and (3) HIV impacted men who indicate a greater degree of spirituality will experience less psychological distress than those who possess lower levels of spirituality.

METHOD

Participants

A total of 100 males infected with HIV agreed to participate in this research project. All male volunteers were solicited from the Human Retroviral Disease (HRD) clinics of a large, Mid-western medical center. Patients who receive services from this facility are typically from the inner-city and are generally economically challenged and without health insurance.

Recent demographic information for men attending these clinics indicates the following racial composition: 76% African-American; 15.8% Latino; 7.5% Caucasian; and .7% Other. The age range of patients in the HRD clinics is young adulthood to senescence with a majority of patients ranging in age between 21-35 years. By and large, these patients are economically challenged whether by income, lack of health insurance, or both.

Table 1 contains relevant information regarding demographic information, sexual orientation, sexual activity, and disease status of the participants.

As shown in Table 1, the majority of the participants were between 30 to 40 years of age. The mean age of the participants was 36.80 years ($SD = 7.73$), and participants ranged in age from 22 to 58 years. The sample was 69% African-American, 12% Latino and 15% Caucasian which approximately parallels the ethnic/racial proportions of men who attend the HRD clinics at the facility.

There were no significant differences among African-Americans, Latinos, and Caucasians across the following variables: age; educational level; length of time diagnosed with HIV (in months); degree of perceived connectedness with a religious organization; and current employment. The number of reported physical symptoms did significantly differ across ethnic-racial status, $[F(2,91) = 6.15, p < .003]$. A Scheffe Multiple Range test which incorporated the calculation for harmonic N due to disparate group sizes was utilized to examine underlying group differences. This analysis revealed that Latino males had a significantly greater number of physical complaints ($M = 7.17$,

TABLE 1. Information Regarding Demographics, Sexual History, and Disease Status

Characteristic	Frequency	Characteristic	Frequency
Age		Current Sexual Activity	
< 30 Years	18	Women	33
30 to 40 Years	52	Men	30
41 to 50 Years	24	Abstinence or Self-Sex	30
> 50 Years	6	Both Men and Women	5
		Not Reported	2
Race			
African-American	69	Past Sexual Activity	
Caucasian	15	Men	35
Latino	12	Women	37
Native American	2	Both	25
Other	2	Not Reported	3
Education		Means of HIV Infection	
< 8th Grade	3	Homosex Sex Activity	45
8th Grade Graduate	1	IV Drug Use	18
8th Grade + Some HS	22	Heterosex Sex Activity	15
HS Graduate	17	Blood Transfusion	3
HS + Some College	44	Unspecified Sex Activity	1
Undergraduate Degree	6	Other	1
Some Graduate Educat	4	Unsure	15
Graduate Degree	1	Not Reported	2
Not Reported	2		
		Most recent CD4 count	
Current Employment Status		< 100	48
Not Employed	78	100–200	11
Employed	22	201–500	24
		> 500	12
Religious Affiliation		Not Available	5
Baptist	49		
Catholic	23	Number of symptoms at testing	
Jewish	2	0	8
Other	15	1-3	28
None	11	4-7	38
		8-11	19
Sexual Orientation		12-14	5
Homosexual	41	No Response	2
Heterosexual	40		
Bisexual		Health Status	
Not Reported	17	HIV+ (non-AIDS)	31
	2	AIDS	67
		Undetermined	2

$SD = 4.50$, $n = 12$) than did African-American males ($M = 4.14$, $SD = 2.91$, $n = 67$), $p < .05$.

Information regarding sexual history indicated there was almost identical representation between groups of men reporting a homosexual (41%) and heterosexual (40%) sexual orientation. In this sample of 100 men, 67% were medically diagnosed with AIDS. Most recent CD4 counts indicated that 59% of the participants had CD4 counts below the 200cmm mark and 12% had CD4 counts above 500cmm. Five percent of the volunteers had no available CD4 counts but were medically diagnosed with AIDS. The median CD4 value for the group was 95.00cmm along with a mean value of 218.27cmm ($SD = 218.27$cmm). On a checklist of 14 HIV/AIDS related symptoms, participants possessed a mean of 4.99 current symptoms ($SD = 3.49$). A significant percentage of the participants (45%) indicated they believe they contracted HIV through homosexual sexual activity, while 18% and 15% believe they contracted the virus through IV drug use and heterosexual sexual activities, respectively.

MEASURES

The Methods of Coping Inventory (MCI; Namir, Wolcott, Fawzy, & Alumbaugh, 1987) was designed to evaluate how persons with AIDS (PWAs) cope with a diagnosis of AIDS. In particular, the researchers were interested in observing the behavioral and cognitive coping styles PWAs use in managing their illness. The inventory consists of 47 items and takes approximately 15 minutes to complete. A respondent evaluates each item within the context of the following prefacing statement: "Which of these things have you used to help you deal with your diagnosis of AIDS?" Because not all individuals in the current study had AIDS, the leading question was altered to read as follows: "Which of these things have you used to help you deal with your HIV illness?" An individual responds to each item by assigning a value ranging from 1 (never) to 5 (always). The possible range of cumulative scores for each of the types of coping methods is as follows: Active-behavioral coping method–20 to 100 points; Active-cognitive coping method–16 to 80 points; and Avoidance coping method–11 to 55 points. In determining which coping style was a given respondent's primary coping method, mean score values for each type of coping method were computed. The scale with the highest mean value was deemed that individual's primary mode of coping.

After deriving the three supraordinate classes of coping methods (i.e., active-behavioral, active-cognitive, and avoidant), Namir and her colleagues analyzed the three coping methods and derived eight sub-classes of specific coping strategies. These sub-classes of coping strategies are more narrow in definition and convey a more specific type of behavioral and/or cognitive element. Four of the eight coping strategies consist solely of items from only one type of general coping method; however, the remaining four coping strategies collapse across behavioral, cognitive, and/or avoidant coping methods. Their method of analyzing and factoring out these groups is not evident; however, they do provide item lists for each coping strategy and measures of internal consistency using Cronbach's alpha. The eight subcategories of coping strategies along with their alpha values include (1) Active-positive involvement – .90; (2) Active-expressive/information seeking – .88; (3) Active-reliance on others – .86; (4) Cognitive-positive under-standing/create meaning – .66; (5) Cognitive-passive/ruminative – .63; (6) Distraction – .66; (7) Passive resignation – .81; and (8) Avoidance-solitary/passive behavior – .80.

The Spiritual Well-Being Scale (SWBS; Ellison, 1983) was utilized to assess the quality and degree of respondents' spiritual well-being. The SWBS attempts to measure two different facets of spirituali-ty–religious well-being (RWB) and existential well-being (EWB). As conceptualized by Ellison and Paloutzian, RWB addresses the vertical dimension of spirituality (i.e., one's relationship with God), whereas EWB addresses the horizontal dimension of spirituality (i.e., how well an individual relates to his surroundings including community and self). The measure is composed of 20 Likert-type formatted items. Both subscales of the SWBS are comprised of 10 items each. For each response choice a respondent selects his/her choice by circling a value 1 (strongly disagree) to 6 (strongly agree). Scores range from 10 to 60 on both subscales. Additionally, the scores from the RWB and EWB subscales may be combined to derive an overall index of spiritual well-being (SWB) with scores ranging from 20 to 120. Test-retest reliability for the RWB subscale is reported as .88, .73 for the EWB, and .82 for the composite SWB. The SWBS takes approximately 5 minutes to complete.

The Profile of Mood States (POMS; McNair, Lorr, & Droppleman,

1971) is a 65-item, 5-point adjective rating scale commonly used to identify affective mood states and mood changes. It takes five minutes to complete and delivers scores that are amenable to statistical and clinical interpretation. There are six mood factors which are tapped: Tension-Anxiety; Depression-Dejection; Anger-Hostility; Vigor-Activity; Fatigue-Inertia; and Confusion-Bewilderment. In addition to the six mood factor scores, the POMS also provides an overall Total Mood Disturbance (TMD) calculation. The respondent is asked to assess how much of a particular mood state has been experienced during the past week, including the day the scale is completed. Reliability for the POMS was determined by calculating coefficient alpha by means of the Kuder-Richardson-20 formula. The standardized item alpha for the POMS is reported to be .86 by the authors. Test-retest reliability for the measure is reported at .66, and concurrent validity is related to be .80 in comparison to clinical assessment (McNair, 1971).

The Symptom Checklist (SC) was designed specifically for this project and enumerates the 14 most common physical symptoms indicative of HIV infection as identified by the CDC in 1992 (Hultz, Chavez, Williams, & Thomas, 1992). Respondents are asked to place a check-mark next to each symptom they are currently experiencing. The number of reported symptoms are summed to provide a total symptom score.

The Demographic Questionnaire (DQ) was designed specifically for this project and it includes questions regarding age, ethnicity/race, sexual orientation, education, employment, drug use, perceived method of HIV infection, past psychiatric illnesses, and various items assessing sources of social and emotional support. The DQ takes approximately 10 to 15 minutes to complete.

Information gleaned from participants' medical records was used to determine the health status of respondents for purposes of assigning them to one of three possible health status groups. The three classes include men with AIDS, men who are HIV+symptomatic–non-AIDS, and patients who are HIV+asymptomatic–non-AIDS. The health status of participants was determined by following the proposed guidelines for diagnosing AIDS as suggested by the Centers for Disease Control (Hultz et al., 1992). An individual was diagnosed with AIDS when he had a CD4+ T-lymphocyte cell count (CD4 count) of less than 200 per cubic millimeter of blood. An average CD4 count for

adult males is 800 to 1200cmms. In addition to the 1992 CDC guidelines, an AIDS diagnosis was also given (regardless of CD4 count) if
an individual tested as HIV positive and had any of the 23 diagnosti-
cally significant diseases including pneumocystis carinii pneumonia,
candidiasis, mycobacterial infections, wasting syndrome, CMV retinitis, crypto-sporidiosis, toxoplasmosis, and Kaposi's sarcoma and other
cancers, pulmonary tuberculosis, recurrent pneumonia, and invasive
cervical cancer. Information regarding participants' medical diagnoses
and CD4 counts were obtained from medical records; consequently, an
individual who had a CD4 count of below 200 and/or had one of the
above stated diseases indicative of AIDS was classified for this project
in the group of respondents with AIDS. An individual was classified
as HIV+symptomatic if he was not diagnosed with AIDS, but was
positive for HIV and presented with one or more HIV related symptoms (e.g., night sweats, swollen glands). The final group consisted of
HIV+asymptomatic individuals; that is, individuals who were HIV
infected but did not have any HIV related symptoms.

PROCEDURE

Participants for this study were recruited from HRD clinics of a
large Mid-western medical center while they were waiting in the clinic
for an appointment with HRD staff. Subjects were recruited using two
techniques. Flyers and posters (presented in English and Spanish)
were placed within the HRD clinics informing individuals of the research project and the manner in which they could contact the researchers if they were interested in participating in the study. In addition, the lead author (a Caucasian male) made verbal announcements
regarding the project and the need for volunteers to individuals waiting in the lobby of the HRD clinic. The announcements were similar
to the information presented in the flyers and posters. Subjects were
informed that their participation would in no way affect their services
from the HRD clinic and that they were free to discontinue their
participation in the study at any time without consequence. Potential
subjects were told that in return for their participation they would
receive five dollars in compensation. Individuals agreeing to participate in the study were requested to sign a combined written consent
and release of information form. Written consent indicated a volunteer's understanding of and willingness to participate in the study. A

release of information was requested in order to give the researchers permission to review the volunteer's medical records to secure their CD4 counts and medical diagnoses.

After acquiring written consent and release of information approval, each participant received a packet of research measures. Participants completed the questionnaire packets in the waiting area of the clinic while a member of the research team was available to answer any questions. Participants were told not to place their names on the questionnaire packet in order to protect their confidentiality. Each questionnaire packet was prepared with the Symptom Checklist and Demographic Questionnaire occurring last in order of presentation, with the remaining instruments arranged in various orders to counteract the possibility of ordering effects.

RESULTS

A series of Analyses of Variance (ANOVA) and Chi-Square analyses were conducted to determine if there were significant differences in the primary type of coping method utilized by the participants based on their demographics. No significant group differences were found related to age, perceived religious affiliation, time diagnosed with HIV, time diagnosed with AIDS, available social support, number of physical symptoms, educational level, sexual orientation, health status, or racial/ethnic status regarding primary coping method.

Utilizing Namir et al.'s (1987) classifications, the primary coping strategies of the participants were as follows: active-cognitive N = 81; active-behavioral N = 8; and avoidant N = 6. It was hypothesized that HIV infected individuals who primarily utilize active-behavioral coping methods would experience lower levels of psychological distress than their counterparts who primarily utilize avoidance coping strategies. Analyses of Variance were conducted to determine if significant differences were present between the three groups on their scores from the POMS. The results indicated that Total Mood Disturbance (TMD) $[F(2,92) = 3.88, p <.05]$ and Depression $[F(2,93) = 3.76, p <.05]$ scores varied as a function of coping method; however, no statistically significant differences were detected among the other subscales of the POMS. Scheffe Multiple Range Tests using a harmonic N to account for disparate group sizes revealed that individuals who primarily used active-cognitive coping methods tended to have lower TMD

(*M* = 79.95, *SD* = 41.66) scores as compared to participants who primarily utilize avoidance coping methods (TMD, *M* = 125.17, *SD* = 36.62;).

To examine the role of marginalized group status, analyses were also conducted to determine if significant differences among levels of psychological distress were present as a function of sexual orientation. These analyses revealed statistically significant results for TMD [*t* (96) = −2.46, *p* < .02]; and Tension [*t* (96) = −2.58, *p* < .01] scores, and a statistical trend for Depression scores [*t* (96) = −1.88, *p* = .06]. Heterosexual males possessed higher levels of overall psychological disturbance (*M* = 98.20, *SD* = 43.48, *n* = 40) as compared to their homosexual/bisexual counterparts (*M* = 76.71, *SD* = 41.05, *n* = 56). Furthermore, heterosexual males reported higher levels of anxiety (*M* = 1.93, *SD* = .91) as compared to their homosexual/bisexual counterparts (*M* = 1.44, *SD* = .92).

To further explicate the relationship between psychological distress and membership in marginalized groups, analyses of variance were conducted to examine participants' scores on the POMS to determine if affective well-being varied across ethnic/racial group status (i.e., African-American vs. Latino vs. Caucasian). No significant differences were found between the three groups on any of the scores from the POMS; however, when exploring the relationship between ethnic/racial status and psychological distress among homosexual and bisexual participants significant differences were found. Results indicated significant differences in TMD [*F*(2,50) = .4.74, *p* < .01], Depression [*F* (2,51) = 3.64, *p* < .05] and Tension [*F*(2,51) = 3.51, *p* < .05] scores as a function of ethnic/racial status for homosexual and bisexual respondents. Using a Scheffe Multiple Range test with a Harmonic N to detect group differences, homosexual and bisexual Latino respondents reported greater levels of overall psychological distress (*M* = 124.00, *SD* = 41.27, *n* = 5) as compared to their African-American (*M* = 70.32, *SD* = 32.00, *n* = 43) and Caucasian (*M* = 64.00, *SD* = 66.69, *n* = 5) counterparts, *p* < .05. No significant differences in TMD scores were found between African-American and Caucasian homosexual/bisexual males. Homosexual and bisexual Latino participants also reported greater levels of depression (*M* = 2.01, *SD* = .89, *n* = 5) as compared to their Caucasian homosexual/bisexual counterparts (*M* = .56, *SD* = .89, *n* = 5).

It was also hypothesized that overall psychological distress would inversely correlate with overall spiritual well-being. To assess this hypothesis, a series of Pearson Product Moment Correlations were conducted between spiritual well-being (i.e., religious, existential, and overall spiritual well-being) and subscale measures of psychological distress. The results indicated that each correlation between the different components of spiritual well-being and psychological distress were significant. In each instance the direction of the correlation was inverse with the exception of the significant correlation between Vigor subscale scores and the three measures of spiritual well-being. Significant results are presented in Table 2.

Analyses assessing the relationship between spiritual well-being and coping methods were also conducted. Spiritual well-being directly correlated with active-cognitive coping methods [$r(95)$ .30, $p < .01$] and active-behavioral coping methods [$r(95) = .24, p < .01$), and inversely correlated with avoidant coping methods ($r(95) = -.23$, $p < .05$). Collectively, these results suggest that for individuals impacted by HIV, spiritual well-being was associated with the use of active-cognitive and active-behavioral coping methods, and that elevations in

TABLE 2. Pearson Correlations Between Subscales of Profile of Mood States and Spiritual Well-Being

	Spiritual Well Being Scores		
	Religious	Existential	Spiritual
POMS Scores			
Depression	-.32**	-.48**	-.45**
Tension	-.43**	-.46**	-.50**
Confision	-.39**	-.51**	-.50**
Fatigue	-.28**	-.26**	-.30**
Anger	-.28**	-.30**	-.33**
Vigor	.18*	.39**	.30**
Total Mood Disturbance	-.37**	-.46**	-.46**

Note: * = significance at the .05 level
      ** = significance at least the .01 level
      DF = 95

spiritual well-being were generally associated with decreases in the use of avoidant coping methods.

Considering that a number of variables were found to be significantly associated with measures of psychological distress, a step-wise multiple regression analysis was conducted to determine the relative degrees of influence these variables possessed in predicting psychological distress. In this analysis, total mood disturbance was the criterion variable, and the predictor variables selected for analysis included spiritual well-being, avoidant coping method, active-behavioral coping method, active-cognitive coping method, perceived helpfulness of supports, number of physical symptoms reported at time of testing, connectedness to religious group, sexual orientation, and ethnicity/race. The results indicate that spiritual well-being and number of physical symptoms were significant predictors of psychological distress. Spiritual well-being was found to be the primary predictor of TMD scores. In combination, spiritual well-being and number of symptoms accounted for 29% of the variance in TMD scores [$r(80) = .54, p < .001$].

Subsequently, a series of multiple regression analyses were conducted on the various subscales of psychological distress to determine the relative association of spiritual well-being and number of physical symptoms on the various POMS subscale scores. Both spiritual well-being and number of physical symptoms were found to be significantly related to five of the six subscale measures of psychological distress. On the Confusion, Anger, Depression, and Tension subscales, measures of spiritual well-being and number of physical symptoms emerged as significant predictors: Confusion, $r(3,78) = .57, p < .001$; Anger, $r(2,79) = .43, p < .001$; Depression, $r(2,79) = .49, p < .001$; Tension, $r(2,79) = .54, p < .001$. Spiritual well-being and number of physical symptoms accounted for 32% of the variance in Confusion scores, 18% of the variance in Anger scores, 24% of the variance in Depression scores, and 29% of the variance in Tension scores. As in the overall analysis of total mood disturbance, spiritual well-being and number of physical symptoms were relatively similar in weighted power of prediction with the greatest predictor of the four subscale scores being spiritual well-being. On the Fatigue subscale, only number of physical symptoms significantly predicted fatigue scores, $r(1,80) = .33, p < .01$. None of the predictor variables included in the multiple regression analysis significantly predicted outcomes on scores for the Vigor subscale of the POMS.

DISCUSSION

The findings of this study are similar to those reported by Namir et al., (1987) in that men who primarily engage in avoidant coping behaviors are more likely to have higher levels of overall psychological distress and to report elevated levels of depressed mood when compared to men who primarily utilize an active coping strategy. In their research, they discovered that men who primarily utilized avoidant coping methods reported increased mood disturbance. Additionally, Namir and her colleagues also found that men who primarily utilized active coping methods had increased self-esteem, and displayed a trend towards increased mood. The results of this study indicate that there is a strong relationship between increased positive mood for men who primarily utilize active-cognitive coping methods as compared to men who primarily utilize avoidant coping methods.

The current findings may be explained by assessing the different patterns of behaviors and cognitive styles that are germane to either coping group. For instance, men who indicate a primarily active-cognitive coping style are more likely to reflect upon the positive changes in life since the onset of their illness (e.g., increased closeness in relationships), are more positive in outlook regarding their illness and life (e.g., hope and meaning), and make plans for the future. They also are more likely to reflect upon the meaning of their illness as well as life in general. In effect, it seems that males who primarily engage in active-cognitive coping methods are more likely to integrate their illness into their life experience and create a balanced perspective of the negative and positive aspects that their illness allows; consequently, their level of overall mood disturbance is likely to be relatively low when compared to individuals who tend to primarily avoid confronting their HIV illness.

Avoidant copers are more likely to suppress and avoid thoughts and feelings related to HIV illness (Namir et al., 1987) which can function to increase the level of overall mood disturbance in a number of ways. First, avoidant coping methods require a great deal of psychological energy to keep unpleasant thoughts and feelings out of conscious awareness. Second, avoidance often leads to a distancing from significant sources of social/emotional and medical supports which can further translate into feelings of isolation, helplessness, hopelessness, and despair. Third, avoidance may lead to an increase of substance use which can engender a number of psychological and social problems.

The findings of this study also indicate that age, race, religious affiliation, educational level, length of time diagnosed with HIV infection or AIDS, availability of social/emotional supports, sexual orientation, and health status do not differentiate between type of primary coping method. However, the results indicate that level of spiritual well-being strongly differentiates between men who utilize active-cognitive as compared to avoidant coping methods. Men who reported higher levels of religious well-being and existential well-being were more likely to utilize active-cognitive coping methods and less likely to utilize avoidant coping methods. This suggests that males infected with HIV who are primarily active-cognitive copers are also likely to experience higher levels of overall spiritual well-being. As Carson et al. (1990) have pointed out, increased spirituality allows an individual to examine life's meaning and mortality with more positive regard and hope for some form of continued existence. Hence, spirituality may alleviate disturbances in affect by providing hope and meaning for an individual contemplating personal mortality (Tomer, 1994; Wong, 1994). When spirituality is low, the task of self-observation in the face of impending death can be affectively devastating and thus lead to avoidance as a means to stave off negative affect.

Given that elevations in positive affective functioning are strongly associated with increased spiritual-well being and active-cognitive coping behaviors, males infected with HIV may benefit from interventions that incorporate spiritual components that address religious or existential concerns related to HIV illness. This may be particularly true for African-American and Latino males infected with HIV due to the relative significance that spirituality, the church, and religion play in their cultures (Cervantes & Ramirez, 1992; Nelson, 1982). Church-based support groups might serve as a positive source of support for ethnic/racial minority men living with HIV; however, given the stigmatization of homosexuality and HIV illness within many church communities (Crawford, Allison, Robinson, & Hughes, 1992), the formation of these groups is likely to require additional community intervention. These findings also imply that active, cognitive coping may be an effective mechanism for enhancing mood and providing

HIV impacted clients with feelings of mastery and control in their lives (Gluhoski, 1996).

For this sample of 100 men, there was no detectable association between the use of active-behavioral coping methods or derivative behavioral coping strategies and levels of psychological distress. These findings are quite different than those of Namir and her colleagues (1987), Feifel (1987) and Wolf (1991). In general, this research suggested that active-behavioral coping methods were positively correlated with self-esteem and inversely correlated with mood disturbance. What is important to note is that the participants in those studies were primarily gay, Caucasian males. The racial composition of their study is starkly different from the present study and coupled with the current findings the psychologically healthy implications of active-behavioral coping methods may not generalize to ethnic/racial minority members.

It can be postulated that increased levels of active-behavioral coping methods are difficult for men in this study for two reasons. First, given that most of the participants of this study were in the later stages of HIV illness, it would seem more difficult for HIV infected males to avoid the finality that HIV/AIDS engenders as well as the subsequent futility associated with attempts to effectively combat dealing with failing health; consequently, increased symptomatology and concomitant depression may lessen the likelihood that an individual will participate in active-behavioral coping methods.

Second, many of the men in this sample are members of marginalized groups (e.g., ethnic/racial minority members, homosexuals, IV drug users, PWAs). As members of socially marginalized groups, they are accustomed to encountering political, economic, and social disenfranchisement from mainstream institutional settings and society. Given their decreased feelings of empowerment, mistrust of institutionalized authorities, and the feelings of futility often associated with HIV disease, behavioral methods of coping may not seem feasible or likely for the men in this study.

Further research is required to address the disparity between the current findings and those of Namir et al. (1987) regarding the association between behavioral coping methods and mood disturbance or psychological distress. Until the relative value of behavioral coping methods in relation to the psychological well-being of ethnic/racial minority members infected with HIV is further clarified, no recommendations for increasing the behavioral coping methods can be made when other factors such as active-cognitive coping strategies and spiritual well-being were clearly associated with feelings of positive affect for the men in this study.

The above findings are also significant when considering the role that psychological distress has on medical compliance and immunological functioning (Antoni, 1989; O'Leary, 1990; Levy & Heiden, 1991). As the results of this study indicate, increased spirituality as well as increased utilization of active-cognitive coping methods are associated with increased levels of positive mood. If spirituality and active-cognitive coping positively influence mood and stress levels, they may also increase immunological functioning (Schlesinger et al., 1989). Hence, decreasing stress by increasing spirituality and active-cognitive coping can positively influence symptom onset and/or symptom exacerbation, especially during the later stages of AIDS (Kiecolt-Glaser et al., 1988).

Because most psychological research on HIV illness has been conducted on primarily homosexual, Caucasian males, it was the intention of this study to examine how HIV illness may affect the psychological well-being of African-Americans and Latinos. A general question addressed by this investigation was in what way does HIV illness differently impact upon levels of psychological distress among ethnic/racial minority men as compared to their Caucasian counterparts.

Results indicated that Latinos who contracted HIV through homosexual sexual activity reported more intense feelings of overall negative mood (e.g., sadness, anxiety) than did their African-American and Caucasian counterparts. There are several reasons why Latinos who contract HIV through homosexual sexual activity may experience greater levels of psychological distress. First, within this sample, Latino men in general presented with a significantly greater number of physical symptoms than did African-American men. An increase in number of physical symptoms indicates increased debilitation and a further progression of the HIV infection which leads to decreases in emotional well-being (Tross et al., 1986). As symptoms become more numerous and evident, it becomes more difficult to deny the impact of HIV illness as well as to deny the onset of deteriorating health that ultimately leads to death (Moynihan, Christ, & Silver, 1988).

The impact of the number of physical symptoms on levels of overall psychological distress as well as depression were further supported by other analyses in this study. In order to determine the combined impact of various factors upon psychological distress, a step-wise multiple regression analysis was conducted. The findings indicated that for overall psychological distress, spiritual well-being was the strongest predictor of psychological distress followed by the number of physical symptoms a participant possessed. Number of physical symptoms was directly correlated with feelings of vigor and inversely correlated with levels of overall mood disturbance, depression, tension, fatigue, confusion, and anger. Physical symptoms can shatter attempts to avoid dealing with HIV illness and also hinder active-behavioral coping methods which generally require energy. The onset or increase of physical symptoms may impede a given individuals ability to sleep, eat, or exercise properly, all of which serve to build energy, and indirectly bolster mood. Additionally, many of the symptoms of AIDS are disfiguring (e.g., Kaposi Sarcoma) and often negatively impact upon the body-image and self-esteem of PWAs, which often lead to depression and sadness (Tross & Hirsch, 1988).

Aside from the number of physical symptoms, it may be helpful to also consider the impact of cultural norms and religious values on the disparity of mood disturbance scores between HIV infected Latinos and African-Americans. Latino culture stresses the importance of male machismo which is defined by Diaz-Guerror (1975) as a socio-culturally determined need for males to behave in very masculine ways. Within that cultural context, homosexuality may be deemed the antithesis of machismo, and is therefore rejected and less tolerated as compared to other cultures that do not contain strongly dictated and generally pervasive characterizations of stereotypical masculine behaviors (Friedman et al., 1987). Engaging in behaviors that fall outside the range of what is generally accepted of males in terms of masculinity could lead to realistic fears of social isolation, familial rejection, and subsequently, stress. In a comparison of levels of "gay hassles" between HIV infected Latinos and Caucasians, Capitaine and her colleagues (1990) found that Latinos as compared to Caucasians experienced a significantly greater level of harassment from community members as a result of their homosexuality.

Second, the influence of the Catholic church, which has typically been very clear in its renunciation of homosexuality (Nelson, 1982), is a very influential agent of socialization within Latino cultures, and Mexican culture in particular (Cervantes & Ramirez, 1992). Consequently, the Catholic church has a great deal of influence on shaping the mores and norms of Latino culture, and therefore functions in a parallel fashion to machismo in fostering the rejection of homosexuality.

This is not to say that African-Americans and Caucasians are immune to the homophobic attitudes of mainstream American culture and religious institutions. On the contrary, Nelson (1982) points out that the homophobic attitudes of the Catholic church are similarly represented in Protestant and Jewish faiths. Consequently, given that Protestant sects are very influential in the African-American community, it is likely that African-American men infected with HIV via homosexual sexual activity experience pressures from their respective religious institutions as do Latinos. However, it can be hypothesized that culturally indoctrinated machismo and the vociferous homophobic attitudes of the Catholic church are more intense than similar pressures experienced by homosexual African-American and Caucasian males by their respective cultural and religious influences.

Another interesting finding related to level of psychological distress and sexual orientation was the increased level of distress among heterosexuals as compared to homosexual/bisexuals. That is, when controlling for method of contracting HIV infection and ethnic/racial status, heterosexuals in general tested with more intense levels of emotional distress as compared to homosexual/bisexuals. In an extensive review of the relevant literature, no comparable findings have been reported. The disparity between levels of emotional distress of heterosexuals and gay/bisexuals may be attributed to heterosexual males in the sample finding themselves associated with a disease that society has largely deemed as related to homosexuals and IV drug users (King, 1989). Not having the experience of dealing with the intense stigmatization attributed to a disease that is largely associated with marginalized groups in American society may prove overwhelming and psychologically stressful for some heterosexual men.

In addition, homosexual/bisexual individuals have developed an extensive network of peer support in helping members of their community in dealing with HIV illness and AIDS (Christ, Weiner, & Moynihan, 1986). To date, literature addressing social supports, HIV, and sexual orientation do not adequately address the availability of community based support groups for heterosexuals. It may be that community based avenues for social and emotional support are more numerous for HIV infected men who are homosexual as compared to men who are heterosexual. In an attempt to further understand the dynamics of the relationship between mood and sexual orientation for men infected with HIV, future research needs to further assess factors such as available social support and perceptions of stigmatization and shame that may differentially affect heterosexuals, homosexuals, or bisexuals.

CONCLUSION

HIV infection is disproportionately more common among ethnic/racial minorities as compared to Caucasians in the U.S. Yet, the vast majority of research on the psycho-social effects of living with HIV/AIDS has not focused on this population. This study was an attempt to assess the psychological well-being of HIV impacted African-American and Latino males, and to examine the manner in which they cope with their illnesses. The findings from the study revealed that greater levels of spiritual well-being are correlated with positive mood and feelings of energy. In addition, individuals who primarily engaged in active-cognitive coping methods possessed higher levels of positive affect as compared to individuals who primarily engaged in avoidance coping strategies. Gay Latino males presented as having greater levels of psychological distress as compared to their gay African-American and Caucasian counterparts. This finding was largely attributed to gay Latino males having a greater number of HIV physical symptoms and encountering profound homo-negative attitudes associated with Latino cultural norms and religious beliefs.

As with all applied research, there are several limitations associated with this research. First, the small sample size of gay Latino and Caucasian HIV impacted participants limits the confidence one can place in the results of the study and hinder their generalizability. Participants in this study were also self-selected and not randomly drawn; consequently, the internal validity of the study is threatened (Shaughnessy & Zechmeister, 1994). However, the study provides useful information regarding the psychological experiences of ethnic/racial minorities living with HIV and how they manage their illness, it identifies areas in need of future research, and offers recommendations on how to meet the mental health needs of ethnic/racial minorities living with AIDS.

REFERENCES

Antoni, M. H., LaPerriere, A., Schneiderman, N., & Fletcher, M. A. (1989). Stress and immunity in individuals at risk for AIDS. *Stress Medicine, 7*, 35-44.

Burack, J. H., Barrett, D. C., & Stall, R. D. (1993). Depressive symptoms and CD-4 lymphocyte decline among HIV-infected men. *Journal of the American Medical Association, 270*, 2568-2573.

Carson, V., Soeken, K. L., Shanty, J., & Terry, L. (1990). Hope and spiritual well-being: Essentials for living with AIDS. *Perspectives in Psychiatric Care, 26*, 28-34.

Ceballos-Capitaine, A., Szapocznik, J., Blaney, N. T., Morgan, R. O., Millon, C., & Eisdorfer, C. (1990). Ethnicity, emotional distress, stress-related disruption, and coping among HIV seropositive gay males. *Hispanic Journal of Behavioral Sciences, 12*, 135-152.

Centers for Disease Control and Prevention. (1996). *HIV/AIDS Surveillance Report, 8*, 9-10.

Cervantes, J. M., & Ramirez, O. (1992). Spirituality and family dynamics in psychotherapy with Latino children. In L. A. Vargas & J. D. Koss-Chioino (Eds.), *Working with Culture* (pp. 103-128). San Francisco, CA: Jossey-Bass Publishers.

Christ, G. H., Wiener, L. S., & Moynihan, R. I. (1986). Psychosocial issues in AIDS. *Psychiatric Annals, 16*, 173-179.

Crawford, I., Allison, K. W., Robinson, W. L., & Hughes, D. (1992). Attitudes of African-American Baptist ministers towards AIDS. *Journal of Community Psychology, 20*, 304-306.

Diaz-Guerror, R. (1975). *Psychology of the Mexican.* Austin, TX: University of Texas Press.

Ellison, C. W. (1983). Spiritual well-being: Conceptualization and measurement. *Journal of Psychology and Theology, 11*, 330-340.

Faulstich, M. E. (1987). Psychiatric aspects of AIDS. *American Journal of Psychiatry, 144*, 551-555.

Fiefel, H., Strack, S., & Nagy, V. T. (1987). Degree of life-threat and differential use of coping modes. *Journal of Psychosomatic Research, 31*, 91-99.

Friedman, S. R., Sotheran, J. L., Abdul-Quadar, A., Primm, B. J., Des Jarlais, D. C., Leinman, P., Mauge, C., Goldsmith, D. S., El-Sadr, W., & Maslansky, R. (1987). The AIDS epidemic among Blacks and Hispanics. *The Milbank Quarterly, 65*, 455-499.

Gluhoski, V. (1996). Psychotherapy with dying AIDS patients and their significant others. In I. Crawford & B. Fishman (Eds.), *Psychosocial interventions in HIV disease: A stage-focused and culture-specific approach.* Northavale, NJ: Jason Aronson, Inc.

Hultz, B., Chavez, C., Williams, S., & Thomas, D. (Eds.). (1992, December). *Positively Aware.* (Available from The Test Positive Aware Network, Inc. 1340 W. Irving Park, Box #259, Chicago, IL 60613).

Keicolt-Glaser, J. K., & Glaser, R. (1988). Psychological influences on immunity. *American Psychologist, 43*, 892-899.

Kim, C. R., & Rickman, L. S. (1988). Psychological aspects of AIDS: A case report and review of the literature. *Military Medicine, 153*, 638-641.

King, M. B. (1989). Psychosocial status of 192 out-patients with HIV infections and AIDS. *British Journal of Psychiatry, 154,* 237-242.

Levy S. M., & Heiden, L. (1991). Depression, distress, and immunity: Risk factors for infectious disease. *Stress Medicine, 7,* 45-51.

Maj, M. (1990). Psychiatric aspects of HIV-1 infection and AIDS. *Psychological Medicine, 20,* 547-563.

Markowitz, J., Klerman, G., & Perry, S. W. (1992). Interpersonal psychotherapy of depressed HIV-positive outpatients. *Hospital and Community Psychiatry, 43,* 885-890.

McNair, D., Lorr, M., & Droppleman, L. (1981). *Profile of mood states.* San Diego, CA: Educational and Industrial Testing Service.

Namir, S., Wolcott, D. L., Fawzy, F. I., & Alumbaugh, M. J. (1987). Coping with AIDS: Psychological and health implications. *Journal of Applied Social Psychology, 17,* 309-328.

Nelson, J. B. (1982). Religious and moral issues in working with homosexual clients. *Journal of Homosexuality, 7,* 163-175.

O'Leary, A. (1990). Stress, emotion, and human immune function. *Psychological Bulletin, 108,* 363-382.

Peterson, J. L., Coates, T. J., Catania, J., Hilliard, B., Middelton, L., & Hearst, N. (1995). Help-seeking for AIDS high-risk sexual behavior among gay and bisexual African-American men. *AIDS Education and Prevention, 7,* 1-9.

Schlesinger, M., & Yodfat, Y. (1991). The impact of stressful life events on natural killer cells. *Stress Medicine, 7,* 53-60.

Shaughnessy, J. J., & Zechmeister, E. (1994). *Research Methods in Psychology.* New York: McGraw-Hill.

Siegel, K., & Krauss, B. (1991). Living with HIV infection: Adaptive tasks of seropositive gay men. *Journal of Health and Social Behavior, 32,* 17-32.

Tomer, A. (1994). Death anxiety in adult life-theoretical perspectives. In R.A. Neimeyer (Ed.), *Death Anxiety Handbook: Research, Instrumentation, and Application.* Washington, D.C.: Taylor & Francis.

Tross, S., Holland, J., Hirsch, D. A., Schiffman, M., Gold, J., & Safai, B. (1986). Psychological and social impact of AIDS spectrum disorders. In *Proceedings for the second international conference on acquired immunodeficiency syndrome* (p. 157). Paris, France.

Wong, P. T., Reker, G. T., & Gesser, G. (1994). Death attitude profile revised: A multidimensional measure of attitudes toward death. In R. Neimeyer (Ed.), *Death Anxiety Handbook: Research, Instrumentation, and Application.* Washington, D.C.: Taylor & Francis.

Index

T - #0146 - 101024 - C0 - 234/156/5 [7] - CB - 9780789006943 - Gloss Lamination